Social Care and Black Communities

A review of recent research studies

Jabeer Butt

Kurshida Mirza

London: HMSO

Printed in the United Kingdom for HMSO
Dd302845 9/96 C15 G3397 10170

For Imtiaaz

About the Race Equality Unit

The Race Equality Unit (REU) was set up in 1987 and is now a registered charity in its own right. The REU is an agency promoting better social care for Britain's black communities. We have attempted to do this through training; consultancy; research; publications; workshops and conferences.

The REU has published reports and good practice guides on subjects such as user involvement, child protection, social work and social work education, ethnic record keeping and monitoring.

If you would like to know more about the Race Equality Unit please write to REU, 5 Tavistock Place, London WC1H 9SN, or phone 0171 387 3300.

About the Authors

Jabeer Butt is presently a Researcher/Consultant with the Race Equality Unit. Jabeer has carried out research in academic and local government institutions, as well as voluntary organisations. The second part of his research into social services departments' development, implementation and monitoring of services for black communities was published in 1994 by HMSO: *Same Service or Equal Service?* This has recently been followed by *Taking the Initiative,* co-authored with Adele Jones, looking at child protection services provided by the NSPCC.

Kurshida Mirza is at present a freelance researcher. She has carried out research on various issues, in particular housing and homelessness. Her most recent work includes an investigation of the needs of black elders, as well as developing a guide for implementing anti-racist care management and assessment. She has published widely and was co-author of *Action on Homelessness*, a good practice guide for housing authorities, published by the London Housing Unit in 1992.

Contents

Tables and Figures

Acknowledgements

The authors would like to thank the many people that have contributed to this publication.

Firstly, thanks must go to the Social Services Inspectorate, who commissioned this work. Also to members of the SSI who commented on early drafts, in particular Paul Brearley. Additionally to Jenny Owen who played a part in bringing this work to publication.

Our thanks are also due to others who have commented on various chapters, principally members of the Race Equality Unit management committee.

Additionally, we would like to acknowledge our debt to Margaret Hogan and Rachel Walker for their help with editing, and to Jannette Bryan for her help in typing the many revisions.

Finally, we must acknowledge the many researchers and their respondents whose work is examined in this review.

Jabeer Butt and Kurshida Mirza

Introduction

The growth of interest amongst agencies as to how black and minority ethnic communities are experiencing social care is reflected in the growth in published literature. Central to this growth has been the question of whether black communities are receiving any services that fall under the social care umbrella and, if they are, whether this experience has been supportive.

The fact that the majority of this research is policy (or practice) driven is a reflection of both the origins of this research in the post second World War interest in aiding 'integration' of black communities (Bourne, 1981; Butt 1994b), as well as the desire on the part of black communities to ensure that their needs are met. Clearly, similar comments can be made about 'mainstream' research on social care; however it is particularly important in this context because of the constant presentation of black communities as a 'problem'.

There have been two repercussions. First, there is little research on how black communities have met their own social care needs in the face of failure of traditional agencies to supply services. Second, there is little evidence of black communities playing an active role in setting the research agenda. Malcolm Cross has recently noted:

> One of the major consequences of being a minority in any society is that there is a tendency for others to identify one's problems, as well as the 'solutions' which is thought appropriate and possible to provide . . . Even where we have progressed from the crude assumption that difficulties of integration are caused by an incongruence of cultural values, social and economic policies with a 'race dimension' are often replete with stereotypes that say more about the definers than the defined.

He proceeds to admit:

> It is time for some humility on the part of social researchers themselves. For many years, investigators of all theoretical persuasions and political views have assumed that they *knew* what the issues were. If the agenda for research and action is to be relevant for the 1990s, then it has to be one which is proclaimed by minorities. To those who wish to hear, there are many articulate voices pressing the claims of a myriad of new concerns. It will be our job to listen. (Cross, 1991:311)

To this recognition of the limitation of existing research we must add that much of this literature remains on the margins of the many debates taking place in social care. This reflects the continued failure of the existing research agencies to seriously address black communities' experience of social care (Evandrou, 1994:599), as well as the limited funding of research on black communities.

These criticisms are not presented in order to denigrate the material that is available. But it is important for us to begin the process of developing an analytical framework for understanding the available material, the gaps that exist and what it therefore tells us about the incidence, prevalence and characteristics of social care needs of black communities.

With these caveats in mind, it is nevertheless the case that there is now a set of research studies that can be used to explore the experience of social care of black communities. Therefore, the aims of this review are to scrutinise currently available documents and data-sources which will throw light on the prevalence, incidence and characteristics of social care (and related health) needs of black and minority ethnic communities. In addition, the review will consider and summarise what is known about the take up of and access to social services of ethnic minority communities.

These aims have been translated into the following tasks:

- identify and summarise significant surveys, studies or other research of relevance (mainly published since January 1980);

- collate the main indications of incidence, prevalence and charac-teristics of social care needs of black and minority ethnic groups, structured to relate to main personal social services areas and/or client groups (ie children and families, elders, mental health, dis-ability, carers);

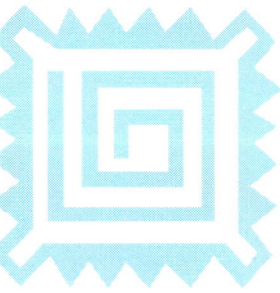

- summarise indications relating to take up and access, delivery and receipt of services and other related matters where appropriate.

Next in this chapter we detail the methodology adopted and then continue with the development of our analytical framework by focus-ing on how we identify needs and the importance of perspectives in research. This chapter concludes with a brief outline of the report.

Terminology

In the context of this review we define black and minority ethnic groups as those people coming from Africa, the Caribbean and Asia and we use the terms 'black people' or 'black communities' as shorthand in the rest of this review. However, where research papers have focused on particular communities, for example 'Afro-Caribbeans', we have highlighted this fact. Furthermore, some authors continue to use negative terms such as 'non-white' (Neill and Williams, 1992; Bebbington and Miles, 1990) or associate the word ethnic only with black and minority ethnic communities (Robson et al, 1995); for the sake of consistency we use these terms too when drawing on these studies. Finally, when discussing issues such as demography and children in care, the terms used do have a particular bearing on the issue and we highlight this in the relevant chapters.

Methodology

We first highlighted the various bibliographies that exist on black communities, in particular those that deal with social care (Johnson, 1985; Atkin and Rollings, 1991; Institute of Race Relations, 1993; Gordon and Klug, 1984; Amin, Fernandes and Gordon, 1988; Shaw, 1988 and 1994). This was augmented by a computer search of all the material held by the NISW library as well as an inspection of the journal New Community. The Race Equality Unit has its own small collection of publicly available material which has not been published, and this was consulted too. A proforma was used to record the abstract for each piece that was read. This proforma also had a pre-coded summary sheet which allowed each piece to be categorised. In addition some effort was put into further analysing the 1991 Census.

Work on the review began in February 1995 and was completed in May 1995. The final draft of this report was produced in October 1995.

Scope of the review
A review examining the social care needs of black communities will inevitably be wide-ranging. Furthermore, existing attempts to review social care needs have often resulted in mammoth tomes, for example Sinclair et al (1990). A similar amount of research is not available with regard to England's black communities (or the United Kingdom's for that matter); nevertheless Atkin and Rollings' (1991) review of some aspects of community care occupied 75 pages.

It was possible, however, to identify some boundaries for this review and necessary because of the limited time and resources available to this project. First, the review focused on studies published since 1980. Second, while identifying datasources that were worth exploring further, the review does not carry out much new analysis of existing data. Third, the review marshals material relating to the experience of black communities mainly in England. However, some of the studies referred to draw material from Scotland, Wales and Northern Ireland, while others do not specify the geographical boundaries of their data collection. It is also likely that there are significant parallels with Scotland, Wales and Northern Ireland in the experience of social care of England's black communities. Finally, the review is about social care needs of black communities and not about black people employed in the social care sector.

Sources for the review
Sources for the review fall into three categories: (a) academic or published research; (b) local authority studies that are available to the public; (c) voluntary and community group studies.

The necessity of using these three sources is dictated by two factors: the comparatively limited attention paid to black communities by mainstream research; in addition, the need to account for voices that have not always been given an opportunity by those involved in researching black communities. In general there is sometimes an exaggerated value attached to some academic research (particularly that of epidemiological and statistical origin) while not enough attention is paid to the work of local authorities and voluntary and community groups. Equally, small-scale localised studies must be treated with care and their unique nature makes it difficult to generalise from these.

Gaps in the review

There are a number of gaps in this review: for example we make little reference to black communities' experience of HIV and AIDS and the social care needs that arise out of these experiences. Some of the gaps owe as much to idiosyncrasy as to the relevance or quality of the material not covered: for example a literature now exists on the experience of black young people leaving care. However, some of the gaps are due to pressure on resources and the need to cover such a disparate literature in a very short time scale; while others are due to the lack of information available: for example studies on elder abuse or the comparative costs of community care packages.

To counter some of these gaps we have attempted to ensure as extensive a list of references as possible, so those wishing to explore areas not covered by this review are able to do so.

Methodology of the studies reviewed
It is difficult to discuss conclusions without drawing attention to some methodological issues. Firstly, there are very few national studies and almost none that cross national boundaries. National studies that have focused on particular issues (for example hospital discharge) rather than the experience of particular communities, have often not referred to black communities or done so only in passing (Levin,

Moriarty and Gorbach, 1994), or done so as an afterthought (Rowe at al, 1989).

The lack of national studies is not only problematic in itself, but also because it makes it difficult to assess how unique local studies are. Clearly, the weight of local studies on some issues (for example black elders, or children in care) means that we can make a strong argument that together the findings do provide a national not just a local picture. Nevertheless, doubts will persist and more weight will be attached to the national studies that mention black communities briefly (for example Bebbington and Miles, 1989) than local studies that have explored the issues in an in-depth way (for example Barn, 1993).

A further difficulty to be noted is the rigour with which the classifying of ethnicity has taken place. Firstly, there is a wide variety of categories used, making comparison between studies difficult. Secondly and most importantly, there has been a failure to indicate how ethnicity was assessed and by whom. This seems to be a particular issue for those who have relied on case notes. The outcry that has accompanied past attempts to record ethnicity without asking those whose ethnicity is being assessed (Butt, 1991) should warn researchers of the ethical dangers of this practice. Equally, the sophisticated statistical analysis that this information has sometimes been subjected to requires a higher order of confidence in the original data than is true for simple descriptive statistics.

These limitations are probably applicable to a lot of social enquiry; however they are particularly important in an area of enquiry which is racked with both political and practice based controversy. Researchers must make clear how they are collecting this information and readers should perhaps add discussion of how researchers have addressed this question as another measure of the quality of the work being presented.

Interpreting the evidence

Our discussion of the policy driven nature of research on black communities has already suggested the necessity of going beyond the usual critical approach we adopt in interpreting research evidence. How we identify need (or problems) and the perspectives that inform the way we conduct and analyse research are further aspects of the analytical framework we have adopted in considering the evidence of the incidence, prevalence and characteristics of social care needs.

Need analysis

There is a reluctance in both the specific literature on black communities, as well as the more comprehensive literature detailing social care needs of white communities, to discuss: what is a need or what are needs? While the expansion of interest in performance indicators has meant more attention being paid to outcomes of social care interventions, this has not necessarily led to a greater interest in being clear about what we mean by needs (a necessity for evaluating outcomes). This reluctance to deal with a fundamental aspect of the process of developing and delivering services may be a consequence of the consensus that appears to prevail in this literature: needs exist and what is of greater significance is explaining why these needs are being satisfied (identifying good practice) or not (inappropriate or inadequate provision). However, it may also be a consequence of the potentially contentious nature of this debate both in political terms and when discussing the needs of those groups who may have been ignored: women; the disabled; black people (Doyal and Gough, 1991).

McKillip in his discussion of need analysis suggests that 'A need is the value judgement that some group has a problem that can be solved'. He proceeds to unpack this definition by highlighting four aspects:

(1) Recognising need involves values. People with different values will recognise different needs. Further, the person seeing the need and the person experiencing the need may differ. An observer may judge your state of affairs inadequate, even though you yourself experience no dissatisfaction.

(2) A need is possessed by a particular group of people in a certain set of circumstances. A description of the target population and its environment is an important part of need analysis.

(3) A problem is an inadequate outcome that violates expectations. There are many sources of expectations, reflecting different values.

(4) Recognition of a need involves a judgement that a solution exists for a problem. A problem may have potential solutions, solutions that vary in the probability of alleviating the problem, and in the cost and the feasibility of implementation. (McKillip, 1987:10)

McKillip explores the third aspect of his definition further. He suggests that 'Problems are recognised by comparison with expectations for what can or ought to be'. He proceeds to summarise the work of Bradshaw (1972) in identifying four types of expectations:

- normative need: expectation based on an expert definition of adequate levels of performance or service;

- expressed need: expectations are indicated by use of services;

- felt need: expectations that members of a group have for their own outcomes;

- comparative need: expectations are based on the performance of a group other than the target population (McKillip, 1987:11-12).

The likelihood that often these four types of expectations intermingle in reality does not negate the value of McKillip's (and Bradshaw's) analysis in helping us to think about needs. Its immediate value is that it helps to categorise the studies that are referenced in this review. Many of the studies identify need in terms of normative need (Fratter et al, 1991 for example). In addition some will combine normative need with expressed need (Askham et al, 1995 for example) while others will combine normative need with comparative need (Barn, 1993 for example). In terms of comparative need per se, research on black communities has been particularly criticised for the failure to do this regularly (Williams, 1990). However, this criticism could equally be levelled at 'mainstream' research (Butt, 1995). More importantly, few of the studies tackle felt need and therefore it is not surprising to find a limited number of studies originating in a user perspective.

McKillip's analysis also makes clear the role of values in need analysis and the identification of solutions, and here the history of social care provision to black communities could be used as case example. Social care provision to black communities has gone from the colour blind (or assimilationist) approach, to the multi-cultural (pluralist) approach, to the anti-racist approach. The first approach suggested that where needs did exist they were the same as those of white communities and therefore there was no need to change services. The second suggests that black communities do have the same needs but that culture is the barrier to accessing services and therefore change focused on gaining cultural knowledge (Roys, 1988; Butt, Gorbach and Ahmad, 1991). The final approach suggests that black communities' needs are possibly different but that these originate from the experience of racism and may require a significant change in practice and in the services we provide (Husband, 1991; Butt, 1994).

Understanding the role played by values in defining needs not only aids the categorisation of studies reviewed here, but can also contribute to our understanding of some of the controversies that have arisen in research on social care and black communities. Examples include the family placement of black children, where it appears that the values you use to define needs will dictate your position on whether black children need to be placed with black families.

Mainstream research

A salient feature of the majority of the studies of social care needs has been their failure to identify whether black people were part of the study (Parker and Lawton, 1994), and if they were whether their experiences were different or not (Lazelle and Lamb, 1994). On the few occasions when black people or communities are referred to, their needs are seen as 'special' (for example Sinclair et al, 1990). This point is further illustrated by local and central government's continued reference to the special needs of black communities: for example funding for black housing associations comes from a 'special needs housing' grant.

There are two consequences of this presentation of the specific needs of black communities as special: first, there is an assumption that we all have basic needs and that black communities have special needs that are over and above these; second, black communities tend to be mixed with other client groups such as disabled or older people. The end result is that black communities have often been seen as being deviant or demanding more than what is available to the white majority communities (Atkin and Rollings, 1993:70), or there is a failure to recognise that there are a number of black client groups whose needs must be met: black disabled people; black older people; black disabled women.

The approach we adopt when considering the issue of need is to always talk of the specific needs of black communities. Just as white communities have specific needs, so do black communities. As importantly we see the needs of black communities as just one facet of the spectrum of needs that social care agencies must respond to.

Research perspectives

Much social care research carried out persists in presenting the researcher and the research tools as neutral, even though there have been significant critiques of both research in the natural sciences and that which falls under the umbrella of the social sciences. Research in the social sciences has come in for particular attention from those committed to promoting anti-oppressive perspectives. An early critique was provided by feminist researchers (Stanley and Wise, 1983) but equally strong criticism has come from those looking at the experiences of black communities (Bourne, 1981; Lawrence, 1982; Mama, 1990) and more recently, the disability movement (Disability, Handicap and Society, Special Issue 1992). Some have attempted to synthesise these critiques and have talked about a new paradigm for research, sometimes described as 'emancipatory' research. Mike Oliver writes:

> Bourne suggests three ways in which this new research paradigm can make a contribution to the combating of racism: (i) a description of experience in the face of 'academics who abstract and distort black experience (however unwittingly)'; (ii) a re-definition of the problem; and (iii) a challenge to the ideology and methodology of dominant research paradigms. To that list written more than 10 years ago, disabled people would want to add the following: (iv) the development of a methodology and set of techniques commensurate with the emancipatory research paradigm; (v) a description of collective experience in the face of academics who are unaware or ignore the existence of the disability movement; and (vi) a monitoring and evaluation of services that are established, controlled and operated by disabled people themselves. (Oliver, 1992)

While much of this debate is about establishing an agenda for present and future research, it inevitably suggests the need to approach completed research from a critical standpoint. Furthermore, it suggests a standpoint that also comments on whether and how black communities have been involved in the research process. It highlights, too, the contentious nature of some of the research on black communities and the role of racism in dictating the research agenda.

Structure of the report

This review has six chapters in addition to the introduction and the conclusion. The chapters are: (2) demography; (3) children and families; (4) black elders and community care; (5) mental health; (6) disability; (7) carers. Chapter two presents the main demographic information on black communities. However, chapters three to seven all have a section highlighting the significant demographic facts relevant to those chapters. In each of these chapters we then attempt to discuss incidence, prevalence, and characteristics of social care needs, as well as access and service delivery.

The conclusion summarises and then draws together the various strands of the review, highlighting some of the emerging themes.

2

Demography

Summary

This chapter examines the burgeoning number of studies exploring various demographic characteristics of England's (and Britain's) black and white communities. The evidence shows that all English local authorities have some black people. However three quarters of black people continue to live in wards where the black presence is higher than the national average, and in some of these wards black people constitute the ethnic majority. The significance of this spatial segregation is that black people continue to live in districts, wards, local authorities where the risk of experiencing deprivation is higher: 22 of 30 authorities with the largest black populations fall within 59 of the 'worst authorities' as identified by the 1991 Deprivation Index.

The evidence further suggests that black communities have grown between 23 to 28 per cent between 1981 and 1991, while white communities have grown by about 1 per cent. Importantly for social care providers this same period has seen the growth of those black people of pensionable age by 168 per cent. For the most part, however, black communities continue to be younger than their white counterparts, with 33 per cent of black people under 15 as opposed to 19 per cent of white people.

The 1991 Census saw the inclusion of an ethnic group[1] question for the first time. This inclusion reflects the growth in availability of a number of national datasets that are analysable by ethnic origin/group: the Labour Force Survey, the General Household Survey, the British Household Panel Study are some examples. The 1991 Census, however, has generated the most significant amount of analysis of this information, from that which was expected (how large are Britain's black communities, where do they live etc), to some which was not expected (whether the level of education of Black and Asian women is associated with them cohabiting [Heath and Dale, 1994:13]). This chapter presents some results from the 1991 Census, as well as other data sources, in order to explore the characteristics of black communities' presence in England (and Britain).

A particular feature of this literature is the use of terms such as 'ethnic minority group' or 'minority ethnic group'. This is both a consequence of the accepted terminology amongst these writers, as well as the impact of the categories used in the 1991 Census which associates the word black principally with those people who originate in the Caribbean and Africa. Unfortunately, some writers continue to use the term 'non-white' to describe all those people who did not describe themselves as white in the 1991 Census. Two points need to be made with regard to our presentation of their analysis in this review: first, these terms such as 'non- white' almost always refer to people of African, Caribbean and Asian origin. Second, as we have done in the other chapters we have used the categories or terms used by the original authors when quoting their analysis.

Significance of numbers

In discussing numbers, a note of caution must be sounded. Often analysis of numbers is used as proxy for identifying need, for example South Glamorgan Social Services Department in their analysis of Census data conclude that Census figures:

> demonstrate for the first time that there are relatively few elderly people from minority ethnic groups in the County's population. While this to a great extent removes the urgency from the need to plan for major service provision for these groups, planning is required to ensure that appropriate services are in place within the next decade; in addition, there remains a need to ensure that appropriate services are available for the relatively small number of people who will need them in the short term. (South Glamorgan County Council, 1994:16)

Robson (1995) and his colleagues, in their production of a matrix of deprivation in English authorities for the Department of Environment (DOE), appear to be involved in a similar process. They wish to provide a mechanism for the DOE to target resources to the most deprived areas. Although they identify the 'close associations' between their measures of the incidence of deprivation with the prevalence of 'ethnic groups' (Robson et al, 1995:82 and Annexe 7), they distinguish between the incidence of deprivation and those who are at higher risk of experiencing deprivation. They note:

> In selecting potential indicators, there are important distinctions between categories of measures. The most significant is between 'direct' and 'indirect' measures; or, more realistically, between measures of the incidence of deprivation (for example, low income, unemployment or ill health) and measure of vulnerable groups with a higher risk of being deprived (for example, pensioners, lone-parent families and ethnic groups) ... Not all members of such groups are necessarily deprived; and those whose deprivation consists, for example, of living in poor housing or of being unemployed would be included in indicators measuring such aspects more directly ... Moreover, the

exclusion of indicators based solely on vulnerable groups avoids
the risk of stereotyping or labelling. (Robson et al, 1995:81)

The temptation to use these statistics to justify or deny the provision
of services is great. This is particularly so as a number of those who
promoted the inclusion of the ethnic group question in the 1991
Census made exaggerated claims as to what the consequence would
be of this information being collected and collated (for example
Brochlain, 1991). However, the value of these statistics lies in the
provision of a description of the target population and the service
environment (McKillip, 1987:8), not in their ability to identify or
quantify need. Therefore, a large number of black pensioners in a
particular area should not necessarily be seen as making service
development more urgent; neither should a small number of black
pensioners downgrade the importance of providing appropriate
services.

Spatial distribution of England's black communities

Teague notes that 'ethnic minorities' accounted for 5.5 per cent of
the total population of Great Britain: around 3.015 million people
(Teague, 1993:13). This figure is higher than the estimated figure of
2.677 million produced by OPCS in the Labour Force Survey 1990
and 91. The reasons for the lower LFS figure go beyond the differing
categories used by the LFS and the 1991 Census. Charlie Owen
suggests that the LFS has consistently under-estimated the size of
Britain's 'ethnic minority' population because of higher levels of non-
participation in this survey (Owen, C. 1993:22).

A further complication in detailing the size of Britain's black
communities is the fact that the 1991 Census missed 1.1 million
people. This would be of little significance but for the fact that non-
response was not uniform across the country (the majority of the
non-response was in inner city areas). In addition, non-response was
greatest amongst men between the ages of 20 to 29. OPCS suggests
that the consequence of this undercounting[2] is that Black Caribbeans
may have been undercounted by 3 per cent, Black Africans by 5 per
cent, Black Others by 4 per cent, and other ethnic minority groups by
similar percentages. In addition men aged between 20-29 from all ethnic groups (including white) may have been undercounted by 15 per
cent (OPCS, 1994).

Of these 3 million people the largest group was Indians who num-
bered around 840 thousand. The second largest of these ethnic
minority communities was Black Caribbeans and they amounted to
around 500 thousand people. The picture for England suggests a
similar pattern, though as Table 1 shows the ethnic minority groups

constitute a slightly larger percentage of the population than for Great Britain as a whole: 6.11 per cent of England as opposed to 5.5 per cent for Great Britain. Table 1 also shows that of the 3 million people of ethnic minority origin in Great Britain, about 2.9 million live in England.

Table 1   Ethnic group of resident population for England

Ethnic group	Male	Female	Total	% of total	% of ethnic minority groups
White	21358956	22785383	44144339	93.81	
Black Caribbean	237217	258465	495682	1.05	17.03
Black African	103685	103233	206918	0.44	7.11
Black Other	84390	87892	172282	0.37	5.92
Indian	414220	409601	823821	1.75	28.30
Pakistani	231785	217861	449646	0.96	15.45
Bangladeshi	82228	75653	157881	0.34	5.42
Chinese	69705	71956	141661	0.30	4.87
Asian Other	89600	99653	189253	0.40	6.50
Other	141103	132618	273721	0.58	9.40
Total	22812889	24242315	47055204	100.00	
Ethnic minority groups	1453933	1456932	2910865		100.00

Source: 1991 Census

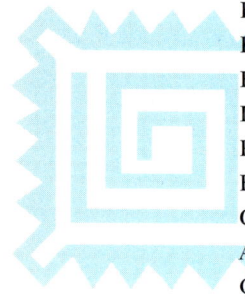

The larger presence of black communities in England is a facet of the spatial distribution of black communities. It has long been accepted that black communities have congregated in particular conurbations (Population Statistics Division, 1986:19). The likelihood that this may mean black communities constitute a significant proportion of the catchment of some social work teams, even though this is not true for their social services department as a whole, has also been acknowledged. Further, Butt, Gorbach and Ahmad have shown, through analysis of the 1981 Census, that there are as many black people living in county council areas as there are living in metropolitan districts (Butt et al, 1991:15).

The need to use a proxy measure for the number of black people up until 1991 (those people resident in households whose head of household was born in the New Commonwealth or Pakistan) meant that it has been problematic to explore spatial distribution of black people much beyond local authority district level. The potentially more rigorous nature of the 1991 Census means that a number of people have analysed spatial distribution further.

Bailey shows that while 5.5 per cent of the population of Great Britain belongs to an 'ethnic group other than white', in 305 (out of a total of 459) local authority districts these communities constitute less than 2 per cent. In fact, in 211 of these districts the 'non-white' population constitute less than 1 per cent (Bailey, 1993:8). A similar picture emerges when we look at the English local authority districts in isolation. Forrest and Gordon note that of the 366 English local authority districts more than a third have less than 1 per cent of the population from 'minority ethnic groups'. They note:

> Typically, these localities are resort and retirement areas, remoter rural areas and mixed urban/rural, although they also include places such as Chesterfield (0.2%), Derwentside (0.4%) and Bolsover (0.5%). (Forrest and Gordon, 1993:64)

Forrest and Gordon rank all 366 local authority districts according to the percentage of their population from 'minority ethnic groups', noting that Brent is ranked first with 44.80% of its population made up of these communities and the Scilly Isles is ranked 366th, as the only English local authority with apparently no people from minority ethnic groups[3]. They present a map of England showing the spatial distribution of 'minority ethnic groups' and conclude:

> The concentration of minority ethnic groups in London and the Metropolitan areas centred on Birmingham, Manchester, Leicester and Bradford is evident from the map. Of the 20 districts with the highest percentage of the population from minority ethnic groups, 16 are in Greater London. The others are Luton, Slough, Birmingham and Leicester. (Forrest and Gordon, 1993:64)

David Owen (1994 and 1992) has taken the analysis of spatial distribution further in two ways: first, he has desegregated 'ethnic minorities' into the various groupings that the 1991 Census results have been presented in, including an 'Other Other' category; second, he has analysed the data at ward level not just local authority district level. Owen presents a series of maps showing the diversity of distribution of ethnic minority groups, noting for example that the Black Caribbean ethnic group is the most concentrated (in inner and south London and Birmingham [Owen, D, 1994c:24]), while the Chinese community is 'extremely heterogeneous' and does not show the same type of local concentrations as other ethnic minority groups (Owen, D, 1994c:25). Owen's analysis of 10,529 electoral wards and the 'pseudo-postcode sectors of Scotland' lead him to conclude:

> The percentage of the entire population and of white people who live in wards containing no persons from ethnic minority groups at all is very small. However, over three quarters of white people live in wards where the percentage of ethnic minority groups is below the GB average. There is a dramatic contrast with ethnic minority groups, for most of whom the position is

reversed: three quarters of their population live in wards with more than the national average percentage of ethnic minority groups. (Owen, D, 1994d:28)

He continues:

> For Black and South Asian ethnic groups, a notable feature is the large percentage of their populations living in wards where the percentage of the population from ethnic minority groups is more than four times the national average. South Asians are distinctive in having over a quarter of their populations living in wards where ethnic minority groups account for more than 44 per cent of the population, while a small proportion of Indians live in wards where more than 88 per cent of the population are from ethnic minority groups. (Owen, D, 1994d:28)

To summarise, the evidence is clear that there are few areas of England (and Great Britain) where black communities do not have a presence. This is true both in terms of local authority districts but also at ward level. However, for the most part black communities continue to live in areas with higher than average numbers of black people. Once again this is true at the local authority district level, but is particularly so at the ward level. Furthermore, in a number of wards black communities constitute almost half of the local population and in some cases they constitute the ethnic majority group.

These conclusions emphasise the need to ensure that the provision of appropriate services to black communities is on the agenda of all social care providers, as none can claim that this is not a 'problem' for them. More importantly they suggest that for some social work teams or frontline service providers a significant number of the potential client group will be from black communities. The evidence also suggest the need to have a detailed knowledge of local populations because the level of spatial concentration is such that neighbouring wards and districts can have dramatically different populations. Finally, these conclusions suggest that the potential for isolation - where black communities are a small fraction of the size of the white population - is very real.

Change in the size of black communities since 1981

The possible sources of information that allow us to explore change in the size of black communities over time are still limited. The 1991 Census has shown that the use of households whose head of household was born in the New Commonwealth or Pakistan is inaccurate and has become more so with the growth of numbers of black people who were born in Great Britain forming households of their own. Nevertheless Jones, amongst others (Owen, D, 1993d:18; Shaw,

1988), has used the NCWP data from 1980s Labour Force Surveys to suggest that in overall terms the ethnic minority population of Great Britain has grown by about 23 per cent. At the same time the number of white people has grown by about 1 per cent. Owen, whose analysis includes the 1991 Labour Force Survey, agrees with Jones' 1 per cent of growth of white communities but suggests that the growth of the ethnic minority community is nearer 28 per cent (Owen, D, 1993a:9).

Table 2 presents Owen's analysis and shows that there is some diversity in the change between 1981 and 1991 when looking at each of the 'ethnic minority groups'. On this point Owen's analysis concurs with that of Jones, who notes:

> . . . the fastest growing groups within the ethnic minority population are the Bangladeshis and the Africans, whereas the number of Afro-Caribbeans has actually declined. (Jones, 1993:18)

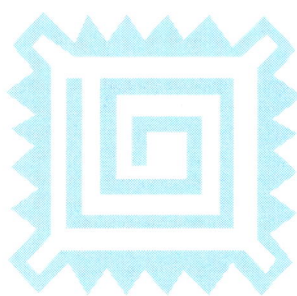

Shaw in his analysis of the components of growth in ethnic minority populations attempted to explore the reason for this growth: was it natural growth (births minus deaths) or net migration (more people coming to Britain then leaving). Shaw demonstrated that two thirds of the annual increase in the period 1984-86 could be explained by natural growth and one third by net migration (Shaw, C, 1988:29). However, Owen suggests that net migration is still a significant factor in explaining the growth in numbers of South Asians (Indians, Pakistanis and Bangladeshis) (Owen, D, 1993d:7).

Table 2   Change in Great Britain's population between 1981 and 1991

Ethnic group	1981 Census	1989-91 Labour Force Survey	Change between 1981-1991	Change as a percentage
White	51000	51808	808	1
West Indian	528	455	-73	-14
African	80	150	70	88
Indian	727	792	65	9
Pakistani	284	485	201	71
Bangladeshi	52	127	75	144
Chinese	92	137	45	49
Arab	53	67	14	26
Mixed	217	309	92	42
Other	60	154	94	157
Not stated	608	495	-113	-19
Ethnic minority groups	2092	2677	585	28

Source: Population Trends 67 and OPCS (1992) as presented by D Owen (1993a:9)

The one ethnic minority group that appears to have declined in size is that defined as West Indian. Beyond noting that net migration for West Indian and Guyanese people totalled only 3.1 per cent between 1980-91, no one has attempted to explain this decline in numbers. However the under-estimation of ethnic minority groups by the LFS and the large number of people who did not state their ethnic group means we need to approach all these figures with some care.

In addition, an examination of the 1991 Census and the responses for Black Caribbean and Black Other suggests a need to be particularly cautious with the data on the community that has its origins in the Caribbean. First, Owen in his analysis contrasts the age profile of those recording themselves as Black Caribbean with those recording themselves as Black Other: Black Caribbeans are older than the other Black groups, while the Black Other group are the most youthful of all ethnic groups (Owen, D, 1993a:3). He further notes that some of the responses may indicate a preference for children born in the United Kingdom to be assessed as Black or Black British rather than Black Caribbean or Black African (Owen, D, 1993a:4), and finally that the majority of Black Other were actually born in this country (Owen, D, 1993a:5). The consequence of this is demonstrated by Table 3, which shows the median age for the Black Other ethnic group as 15.7 years. Put simply, the distinction drawn between Black Caribbeans and Black Others may be understating the size of the Caribbean community because young black people whose parents are from the Caribbean are choosing to describe themselves as Black Other rather than Black Caribbean.

Second, the 1991 Census had two write-in categories (Black Other and 'any other ethnic group') in addition to the 6 pre-coded ones. The coding of the response is detailed in the Appendix. Of particular interest is that the same code was given to those people who described themselves as East African Asians and those who described themselves as Indo-Caribbean, and in presenting the ethnic group results for the 1991 Census these people were categorised as Other Asians. In effect a group that would have been defined as West Indian under the LFS were put in the Other Asian category, possibly leading to a further undercounting of Caribbeans.

To summarise, when it is possible to look at the change in the size of the black communities it is clear that they have grown. The rate of growth in the constituent parts of black communities varies, with the Bangladeshi community growing the most in percentage terms and Pakistanis in actual numbers. Much of this growth is explained by natural growth (more births then deaths) rather than net migration (more people coming than leaving Great Britain), although the latter plays a significant part in the growth of Bangladeshis. Finally, although it appears that the Caribbean community is declining, there is some evidence to suggest we need to be cautious as to how much this reflects a change in the size of the community as opposed to a change in the categories the community chooses to use or analysts choose to place them in.

Age

A striking feature of the presence of black communities in Great Britain has been their 'youth' in comparison to white people. Table 3 presents Owen's analysis of the median ages for all ethnic minority groups derived from the 1991 Census. Figure 1 plots the median ages for men and women for each ethnic group as well as the overall median for the entire population and for all ethnic minorities. The median age of white people is 37.4, but that for all of the 'ethnic minority groups' is 25.5, a difference of over 12 years. The difference for males is 10 years but that for women is over 13 years.

Table 3 Median ages of males and females for all ethnic groups

Ethnic group	All people	Males	Females
White	37.4	35.4	38.9
Black Caribbean	30.2	30.2	30.3
Black African	26.3	26.6	26.0
Black Other	15.7	15.0	16.5
Indian	28.0	28.2	27.9
Pakistani	19.7	19.6	19.7
Bangladeshi	17.0	17.1	16.9
Chinese	28.7	27.9	29.6
Asian Other	30.2	29.2	30.9
Other	21.0	21.6	20.5
Entire population	36.5	35.0	37.9
Ethnic minority groups	25.5	25.3	25.6

Source: 1991 Census as presented by D Owen (1993a:6)

The difference in median age is a result of 39 per cent of white people being over the age of 45, while the 45 plus group only account for around 18.5 per cent of ethnic minority groups. The difference becomes more pronounced if we consider the 65 plus group, who account for 16.9 per cent of white people but only 3.2 per cent of ethnic minorities. Jones states it differently: his analysis of the LFS shows that while 79 per cent of white people are under 60 for 'ethnic minorities', 95 per cent are under 60 (Jones, 1993:23).

Clearly the median age is also impacted on by the percentage of young people and children in particular. The 1991 Census shows that just over 33 per cent of 'ethnic minority groups' are under 15 years

Figure 1 Median ages of males and females of all ethnic groups

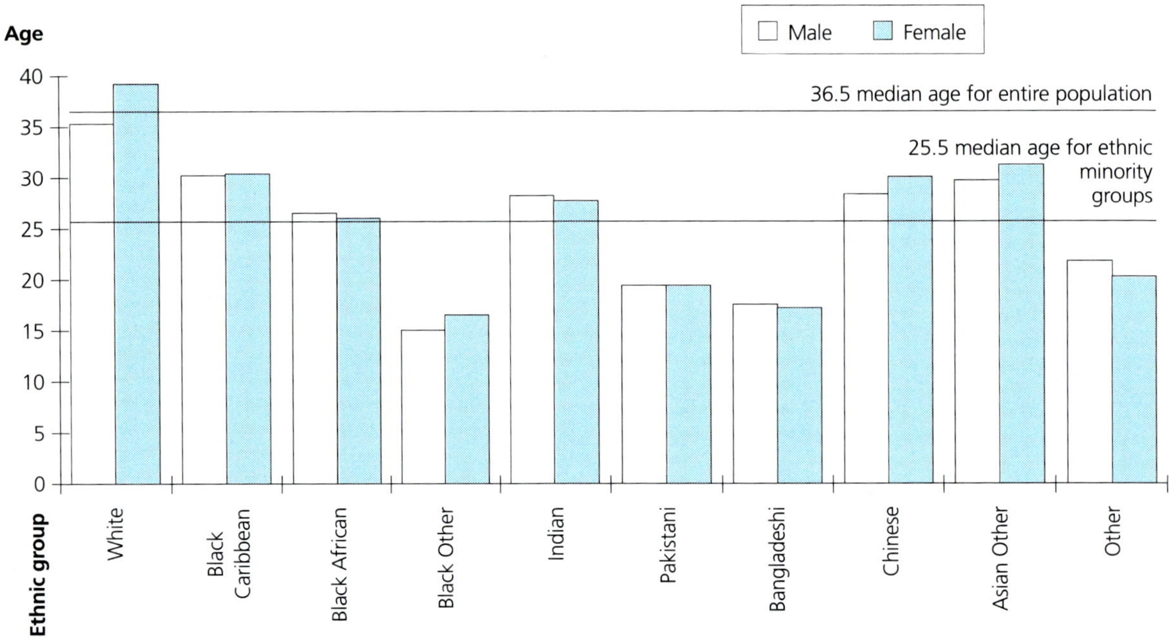

Source: 1991 Census based on analysis presented by D Owen (1993a:6)

old as opposed to just over 19 per cent of white people. The comparatively large number of children in black communities is of interest in itself. It appears to be a product of higher birth rates[4], particularly in the Bangladeshi (47 per cent under 15) and the Pakistani (42 per cent under 15) communities. Taking into account the highly concentrated nature of black communities' presence in Britain, this does suggest that in some areas children from black communities will be in the majority in educational establishments. It also has the consequence that for some time to come black communities will continue to have a younger profile than their white counterparts.

The longer life expectancy of women which sees them make up a larger part of the post-60 population of white people in Britain (and most of western Europe) is not true for Britain's black communities. Firstly, Table 3 shows that while white females have a median age 3 years in excess of their male counterparts, there is little difference between males and females in each of the black communities. When there a is difference in black people it is often men who have a median age in excess of women. Secondly, there appears to be little difference in the number of ethnic minority men and women aged 60 and over. This may be a result of migration patterns, which still means that there are about 104 'ethnic minority' men to 100 'ethnic minority' women (Jones, 1993:24) and therefore there are potentially more men who could survive into the post-60 generation. Fenton has gone as far as arguing that, as a result of migration patterns, men will outnumber women amongst the black elderly (Fenton, 1987:9). However, the 1991 Census suggests equal numbers of male and female black elders rather than more men or more women.

What does appear to be clear is that as a group black elders are likely to grow considerably. Owen details the changes between 1981 and 1991 of various age cohorts and suggests that while the number of NCWP people who are between 45 and pensionable age has grown by 35 per cent, the largest percentage growth has been in those people of pensionable age: 168.6 per cent or from 61,200 in 1981 to 164,306 in 1991 (Owen, 1993a:10).

To summarise, black communities are younger then their white counterparts, with 33 per cent of 'ethnic minorities' under 15 as opposed to 19 per cent of white people. On the other end of the scale over 39 per cent of white people are over the age of 45 as opposed to over 18 per cent of 'ethnic minorities'. This is further demonstrated by the median age for white people being over 13 years in excess of 'ethnic minorities'. The significant number of children in black communities is now being accompanied by a growing number of black people of pensionable age and over. In terms of this group of pensioners, for the most part women do not outnumber men in the post-60 black population, as they do for the white communities.

Households

The disparity in the number of people over the age of 60 is reflected in household structure too. Households with pensioners in white communities account for almost 26 per cent of all white households, while for 'ethnic minorities' groups they account for just over 4 per cent (see Table 4). Of the ethnic minority groups, the largest number of households with pensioners are Black Caribbeans: 7.2 per cent, around 15.5 thousand households. If we exclude the Other category, the Chinese ethnic group have the second largest group of households with pensioners: 3.7 per cent, just under 2 thousand households. The Chinese are followed by Indians who have the third largest group of households with pensioners: 3.6 per cent, just over 8 thousand households. As can be seen by comparing Table 4 with Table 3, these three 'ethnic minority groups' are three of the four groups with the highest median age.

Table 4 also shows the number of lone pensioner households. As is the case with households that have pensioners, white lone pensioner households account for a larger percentage of white households than any of the 'ethnic minority groups': 15.6 per cent as opposed to 2.8 per cent. Of the 'ethnic minority groups' Black Caribbeans have the largest number of lone pensioner households: 5.5 per cent, 11.6 thousand households.

Spatial distribution too differentiates black pensioners from their white counterparts. Forest and Gordon rank the 366 local authority districts in terms of pensioners as a percentage of the total population. They suggest that all the 25 areas with the highest percentage of pensioners are 'classified' as resort or retirement areas or are remoter rural districts (Forrest and Gordon, 1993:41). None of these 25 areas are in the top 50 of Forrest and Gordon's ranked areas in terms of 'minority ethnic groups'.

Owen has suggested that the low percentage of lone pensioner households amongst South Asians (1.5 per cent of all South Asian households), and the comparatively high percentage in ethnic minority groups such as Black Caribbeans and Chinese, may reflect a 'decline in family ties, and the lesser willingness of other ethnic groups to accommodate aged parents' (Owen, D, 1993:6). This appears to be a dubious argument. Firstly, a snapshot survey is being used to assess what is a dynamic relationship: family formation (Heath and Dale, 1994:5). Second, the 1991 Census[5] shows a higher incidence of single adult households and single parent families amongst black groups and Chinese and others in comparison to South Asians (Owen, D, 1993b:5) and therefore it is not surprising that this pattern of households with one adult is carried on into older age.

Table 4   Pensioner households

Ethnic group	Pensioner households in 000s	Pensioners as % of all households	Lone pensioners	Lone pensioners as % of all households
White	5393.6	25.7	3277.6	15.6
Black Caribbean	15.5	7.2	11.6	5.3
Black African	1.5	2.0	1.2	1.6
Black Other	1.3	3.4	1	2.5
Indian	8.1	3.6	4.4	2.0
Pakistani	1.5	1.4	0.9	0.9
Bangladeshi	0.3	1.0	0.2	0.7
Chinese	1.8	3.7	1.2	2.4
Asian other	1.5	2.6	1.1	1.8
Other	4.8	6.2	3.3	4.2
Entire population	5429	24.8	3302.3	15.1
Ethnic minority groups	36.3	4.2	24.7	2.8

Source: 1991 Census as presented by D Owen (1993b:5-7)

Size

Table 5 shows that the number of people per household is higher for all ethnic minority groups than for white people. In overall terms there are 2.43 people per household in the white community, yet there are 3.34 people per household for 'ethnic minority groups'. This is partially explained by the larger number of 'ethnic minority group' households that have three or more adults. However, the more significant factor appears to be the number of children. Jones notes:

> About half of all Bangladeshi and Pakistani households, and about a quarter of African-Asian and Indian households contain large families, compared to 6 per cent of white households. (Jones, 1993:17)

Jones defines large families as 'one or more persons aged 16 or above and three or more under 16; or, three or more persons aged 16 or above and two under 16'. This can be further illustrated through another piece of analysis by Jones: the number of dependent children per family unit (see Figure 2). Jones shows that while the mean number of children per family unit is 0.5 for white people for all 'ethnic minority groups' this figure is 1.0 (Jones, 1993:29).

Table 5   Size of households and the number of adults per household

Ethnic group	Households in 000s	People per household	One adult	Two adults	Three or more adults
White	2102.6	2.43	31.1	52.2	16.7
Black Caribbean	216.5	2.52	44.9	36.4	18.6
Black African	73.3	2.84	41.4	41	17.3
Black Other	38.3	2.51	49.8	40	9.9
Indian	225.6	3.8	12.9	51.6	35.4
Pakistani	100.9	4.81	12.8	51.3	35.7
Bangladeshi	30.7	5.34	10.3	50.9	38.7
Chinese	48.6	3.08	25.6	50.2	23.9
Asian other	59	3.15	23.9	53.2	22.7
Other	77.9	2.74	34.9	49.8	15.2
Entire population	21897.3	2.47	31	52	17
Ethnic minority groups	870.8	3.34	28.2	46.2	25.4

Source: 1991 Census as presented by D Owen (1993b:1)

To summarise, black communities have larger households than their white counterparts (even when desegregated into each ethnic group). This is partially explained by the higher than average number of households that have three or more adults (a possible indicator of the existence of extended families). However, the most important factor appears to be the above average number of children in ethnic minority households/family units.

Figure 2 Mean number of children per family unit

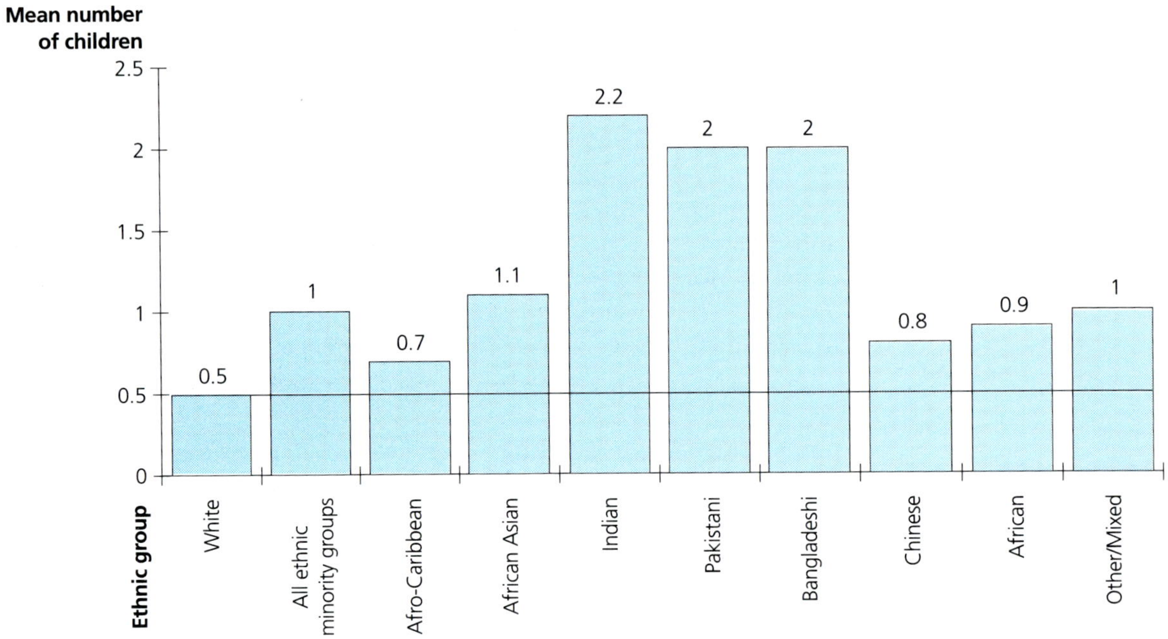

**Mean number
of children**

Source: Labour Force Surveys as analysed by Jones (1993:29)

Although the analysis of household structure emphasises the prevalence of families with children under the age of 16, it also shows the existence of pensioner households. No 'ethnic minority group' has the same percentage of pensioner households or lone pensioner households as white communities do. However, they do appear to exist in most communities and most often for Black Caribbeans, reflecting the earlier arrival of this community to England (Jones, 1993:14).

Housing and tenure

Nationally, 59 per cent of black communities live in accommodation which is owned outright compared to 65 per cent of white people (1988/90 Labour Force Survey). Of those who own their accommodation, large variations within the different black communities exist. For example, 82 per cent of African Asian, 76 per cent Indian and 75 per cent of Pakistani people own their accommodation whilst 46 per cent of Afro-Caribbeans and Bangladeshis own their accommodation. The 1991 Census also shows a similar pattern with a high proportion of owner occupation amongst South Asian people (over three quarters owned their home) compared to the white households (two thirds owned their home) and black groups (just under half own their home). Within each of the minority ethnic categories marked differences in the tenure patterns exist. For example, within the South Asian category, 81.7 per cent of Indian households own their home and the percentage of Pakistani households who are owner occupiers is only slightly less. In contrast, less than half of Bangladeshi households are in owner occupied accommodation.

Renting from the private sector is more common among Pakistani and Bangladeshi households than for white households, and less common for Indian households than for any of the other ethnic groups. The percentage of households renting from housing associations is three times higher among Bangladeshis than for other South Asian or white households. The percentage of households renting from the public sector is only half as high for South Asians as for white households, and is particularly low for Indians. However, 'more than a third of Bangladeshi households live in public sector accommodation, probably because of their relative poverty and concentration in relatively deprived areas such as Tower Hamlets', notes Owen (1994b:8).

Within black groups, all forms of renting are much more common than white households with the public sector being the most common tenure type for Black-Africans. The percentage of households in each of the black ethnic groups renting from housing associations is similar, but private renting is more common amongst Black Africans which, notes Owen (1994a:6), must 'reflect the number of students and refugees in this ethnic group'.

Though a large proportion of black people own their own accommodation there is evidence to suggest that the black community occupy older inner city accommodation, which lacks basic amenities. Furthermore, black households are more likely to experience overcrowding compared to the white population. The English Housing Condition Survey by the Department of Environment in 1976, for example, showed that black communities in general occupied older accommodation and were more likely to lack certain basic amenities and suffer more overcrowding (DOE, 1979a). Indeed the most recent English Housing Condition Survey shows that within the owner occupied sector different ethnic groups occupy different types of housing. For example, households of Asian origin were more likely to own older dwellings: 41 per cent were living in pre-1919 terraced houses compared with 14 per cent of white households (DOE, 1991:104). Similarly, Owen's analysis of the 1991 Census shows that a high level of overcrowding exists within South Asian and black groups compared to white households, with over a fifth of South Asian households having a density greater than one person per

room. Overcrowding for black groups was 7.2 per cent and white
groups 1.8 per cent.

The high levels of owner-occupation amongst black communities,
particularly amongst South Asian people, is a recent phenomenon
and has resulted from the fact that access to other forms of housing
has not been open. For example, Jones (1993) notes:

> The 1974 and 1982 surveys documented the development of
> tenure patterns amongst Afro-Caribbean and South Asian
> people up until the early 1980s. They described the tendency of
> newly arrived immigrants to find housing in the most accessible
> part of the UK housing market, the private rented sector. Once
> they were joined by their dependants and family units were
> established, they needed to find larger and more secure
> accommodation.

However:

> Because of qualifying periods of residency needed to obtain
> council housing, the only option to many immigrants was to buy
> what were often the cheaper properties on the market. In this
> way dramatic differences in both the tenure patterns and the
> quality of housing developed between the South Asian
> population, the Afro-Caribbean population and the white
> population. (Jones, 1993:134)

Furthermore, Jones suggests, that owner occupation for black
communities does not correlate with greater affluence and better
standard housing (as is the case for white people). For example, the
1988/90 Labour Force Survey found that whereas among the general
population the level of owner occupation increases with higher
income, among South Asians owner occupation was 'paradoxically,
most common amongst the lower job levels' (Jones, 1993:134).

Even when black people did find their way into public housing they
often had to wait longer and tended to receive a poorer quality
accommodation compared to white people (Flett et al 1979; Simpson,
1981; CRE 1984a, 1984b, 1989). The Commission for Racial Equality
found evidence of discrimination both in Hackney and Liverpool
(CRE, 1984a; CRE, 1984b). The report on Liverpool stated that
'systematic racial differences exist in the allocation of Council
housing; black people usually have to wait longer for council housing
and when rehoused tend to be given lower quality accommodation'.
Another study (CRE, 1989) found that black households nominated
to housing associations consistently received poorer quality housing.

Social and economic circumstances

Much of the discussion to date has been about the various characteristics of the presence of black communities in England (and Britain). The 1991 Census has also allowed some analysis of the risk of experiencing material and social deprivation. Various approaches have been adopted and while some of these have not focused specifically on the experience of black communities (Forrest and Gordon, 1993:59), others have (Owen, 1994d:28 and Robson et al, 1995:162).

Owen in exploring the question of 'spatial segregation' examined whether ethnic minorities lived in different 'types of areas' to white people, focusing on whether there was any difference in terms of affluence or deprivation. He developed a classification of electoral wards which summarised 21 socio-economic characteristics, and included indicators which covered age structure, household structure, tenure and overcrowding as well as economic characteristics, amongst others. Using these indicators the 10,529 electoral wards (and pseudo-postcode sectors in Scotland) were classified into one of ten area types. After presenting his results in a set of histograms Owen summarised his findings thus:

> The bulk of the population and of the white ethnic group lives in clusters 4, 5, 8 and 9: the traditional industrial areas, suburbs and rural areas. In contrast, most of the ethnic minority group population is found in more highly urbanised environments, though there are fairly dramatic contrasts between ethnic minority groups in the types of residential environment in which they live.

He concludes:

> This analysis demonstrates that the spatial segregation of ethnic groups is accompanied by their social segregation. That is, the types of areas in which ethnic minorities tend to concentrate have very different socio-economic characteristics to those where the bulk of the white population tend to live. (Owen, 1994d:29)

Put simply, there was clear evidence that white people tended to reside in the more affluent wards while ethnic minorities resided in the more deprived areas.

Owen's approach, while successfully demonstrating the accompaniment of residential segregation with socio-economic segregation, adopts a method that has been criticised by those developing indices of deprivation. The criticism is not to do with the inclusion of measures of affluence such as 'entrepreneurship rate', because this is legitimate in terms of the task he has set himself. The criticism is because of his failure to recognise that:

> Not all conditions which are likely to result in deprivation are in themselves forms of deprivation. For example vulnerable groups (such as the elderly or handicapped) should not necessarily be seen as being deprived simply because they have a higher risk of one or more form of deprivation. (Coombes et al, 1995:8)

Owen's inclusion of measures such as the percentage of lone parent families or the percentage of pensioner households are two examples of vulnerable groups rather than the incidence of deprivation.

Following the 1991 Census the Department of Environment (DOE) commissioned two contractors to advise and work on an index which measures levels of relative deprivation across England (Robson et al, 1995 and Coombes et al, 1995). Deprivation continues to pose a major challenge for urban policy in Britain: a key concern is the targeting of assistance on the greatest concentrations of deprivation.

The concept of analysing deprivation is not new. The DOE's designation of Urban Priority Areas using the 1981 Census data has been widely used, not only by government departments, but by other organisations. Despite the controversy over the nature of deprivation, operational definitions and how to measure deprivation (Townsend et al, 1988) the influence of deprivation is now generally accepted (Whitehead, 1987) and the statistical evidence for linking deprivation with ill health, for example, has been established (Townsend et al, 1988).

The DOE report identifies ten issues in its anatomy of deprivation: social environment, physical environment, housing, education, employment, work conditions, income and needs, communications, recreation and health. A correlation of these deprivation indicators with vulnerable groups by enumeration district levels shows that people from 'ethnic [minority] groups' are significantly deprived on each of the indicators. For example, unemployment and ethnicity correlates at .4020 (statistically significant at LE 0.01) and overcrowding at .5948 (statistically significant at LE 0.01). A similar picture emerges at local authority district level and Table 6 reproduces these results.

Using Forrest and Gordon's rankings of authorities with the largest minority ethnic communities and Table 6.3 'Sets of worst authorities' of the 1991 Deprivation Index, we can begin to show what the statistics in Table 6 here mean in reality. Of the 30 authorities with the largest minority ethnic populations, 22 fall within the 59 'worst authorities' as identified by the 1991 Deprivation Index. These authorities are Brent, Newham, Tower Hamlets, Hackney, Ealing, Lambeth, Haringey, Leicester, Waltham Forest, Southwark, Lewisham, Birmingham, Westminster, Wandsworth, Islington, Wolverhampton, Camden, Hammersmith, Bradford, Kensington and Chelsea, Blackburn and Sandwell. The eight that do not are all either outer London boroughs - Harrow, Hounslow, Redbridge, Barnet, Croydon and Merton, or on its periphery - Slough and Luton.

Table 6 Correlations between vulnerable groups and indicators

Indicators	ETHNIC (persons defined as Black or Asian)
UNEMP	
Unemployment, 1991	.4206*
HHA1PR	
Overcrowding, 1991	.8498*
LACKAM	
Lacking amenities, 1991	.4885*
CHILDHG	
Children in unsuitable accommodation, 1991	.0787*
LOERNK	
Children in low-earner households, 1991	.0412*
NOCAR	
No car	.4631*
NOSTUD	
Educational participation, 1991	.4230*
SMR	
Standard mortality rate, 1991	.2068*
MLONGT	
Long-term/Unemployment ratio, 1991	.3315*
INCSUP	
Income support, 1991	.3971*
RATINGH	
Home insurance weightings, 1991	.1874*
LOGCSE	
Low education attainment, 1991	.4982*
DEREL	
Derelict land, 1988	.0892

Source: Robson et al, (1995:162)

To summarise, neither Owen nor the DOE report authors suggest that their analysis of deprivation (or affluence) means that black communities are experiencing deprivation. Jones for example high-lights the 'progress' (Jones, 1993:153) that some ethnic minority groups have made in the labour market, and the DOE analysis shows that in terms of attainment of GCSEs they are not low achievers. However, both Owen and the DOE are clear that these communities live in areas where deprivation is more pronounced. Black communities are at greater risk of experiencing:

- unemployment and this is more likely to be long term;
- overcrowding as well as children living in unsuitable accommodation (even though owner occupation is high amongst groups such as Pakistanis);
- as well as having persons or households living on income support.

Importantly for this review, this evidence suggests that black communities are at greater risk of experiencing some of the stresses so often associated with people who need the services of social care agencies.

Conclusion

The demographic evidence suggests a growing black population in England with significant growth in numbers in one social care client group: black people over 65. At the same time significant numbers of under 16s continue to ensure that black communities have a median age much lower that their white counterparts. Though there is evidence of some movement out of inner London black communities continue to congregate in areas of higher than average numbers of black people. These areas are also often associated with higher incidences of social and economic deprivation.

3

Children and families

Summary

The chapter emphasises the difficulties in comparing and contrasting studies which seem to be different in every way, except for the issues that they are exploring. Nevertheless, the evidence does show that for most black communities, families with dependent children is a common experience and that these families are likely to have more dependent children than their white counterparts. Additionally while evidence presented in other chapters suggests black families are at greater risk of experiencing some of the factors associated with abuse and neglect (poverty for example), there is little evidence of higher rates of abuse or neglect.

The conclusions one can draw about whether black children are over-represented in care are made difficult by some studies drawing their sample from those 'admitted to care' while others drew their sample from those 'in care', amongst other inconsistencies. However all studies agree that entry into care for black children is most likely to occur when they are under five and most suggest that this is more likely to be true of black children than white children. Those studies setting out to specifically explore black representation suggest black children are over-represented. However, national studies suggest any over-representation disappears if controlled for age. An area of agreement across all the studies is the over-representation of children who had one black and one white parent. Furthermore, when studies look at routes of entry they demonstrate that black children are more likely to enter through the voluntary route (Section 2 of 1980 Children Act) than the compulsory route (essentially the 1969 Children and Young Persons Act). But there is disagreement as to whether black children then remain in care under a compulsory legal order.

The studies reviewed here show that once in care black children are more likely than their white counterparts to find themselves placed with families than in residential establishments. This reflects the change in practice which has increasingly viewed family placement as the best option for the care of children. However it has also been the background to the acrimonious debate about the importance of same race placement and in the significance of identity and self-esteem. Rather than re-visiting this debate we explore what evidence there is on the placement outcomes for children. The different measures used by all the studies suggest a need for caution in drawing conclusions. However there is some suggestion that black children placed with black families will share similar (or better) outcomes to white children placed with white families.

Few areas of research on black communities have been without controversy; however the most controversial has been children and families. This is so for two reasons. The first relates to the possible over-representation of black children in the care system. The second is the dominance of the debate on same race or transracial placement of black children. Shaw (1988:89) suggests that this has led to a dominance of this debate in published material also. Importantly, however, most commentators agree that the research on black children and families is lacking. The Department of Health (1991) notes in the context of implementing the sections of the Children Act 1989 which focus on race, religion, language and culture:

> Recent research reports do not provide many suggestions about how this is to be put into effect. Indeed, in many of them ethnic issues are not addressed. None offers data on the dominant issue of whether children must always be placed with families of the same racial background. (DH, 1991:13)

Rowe, Hundley and Garnett (1989) suggest that this lack of research is accompanied by the non-availability of national statistics:

> The current lack of information about black children in care is serious and startling. There are no national statistics and few local studies, even though concern was expressed 20 years ago [1967] about what already appeared to be disproportionately large numbers of black children in the London care system. (Rowe et al: 158)

Ahmad has argued that it is not only that there is a lack of research but that its quality leaves a lot to be desired. She notes:

> It is not necessarily the lack of research that is restricting the acquisition of ethnically sensitive social work skills. Rather it is the methodology and interpretation of research that is mystifying the social work profession to the detriment of black children, young people and their families. (Ahmad, 1989:152)

Echoing Ahmad's criticism, Barn suggests that when research that has been done, it has attempted to explain its findings in terms of the nature of black families:

> Most research studies have immersed themselves in explorations of black family structures and lifestyles, leading some commentators to assert that the black family has been pathologized. (Barn, 1993:16)

Recognising these concerns and having noted some of the limitations of this work, it is still possible to develop a picture of the incidence, prevalence and characteristics of social care needs, as well as explore the provision of services. In terms of this chapter we will focus on households and family structure, child abuse and neglect, black children in the care system, and the placement of children. Juvenile justice, leaving care and private fostering will be mentioned where appropriate.

First, however, it is worthwhile returning to the question of terminology. This is at the heart of some of the difficulties in coming to terms with the evidence, and may cause difficulties in comparing evidence from different studies. The area of most disagreement is around the use of the terms 'mixed origin', 'mixed parentage' or 'mixed race'. Some studies choose to categorise children who have one black and one white parent as black in their analysis (Barn 1993), while others categorise the same group of children as 'mixed race' in their analysis (Bebbington and Miles, 1989) or 'mixed parentage' (Rowe et al, 1989). Others such as Charles et al have developed a more complex form of categorisation in discussing transracial placement (Charles et al, 1992).

The consequences of the differential use of terms is not only the difficulty it creates in comparing studies, but also the possibility that the conclusions that some studies have come to may change if a different form of categorisation is used (see our discussion on page). Without revisiting the original data in all the studies and using standard categories to analyse the data, it is not possible to say how much of the divergence in conclusions of the various studies is due to what was observed, as opposed to how it was categorised. Nevertheless, as we have done in all the other chapters, we continue to use the terminology that the original authors have chosen to use.

Demography

The 1991 Census suggests some variation in the number of households with children under the age of 16 from different ethnic groups. For example, of the white ethnic group 29.5 per cent of families are childless couples while 32.8 per cent of Bangladeshi families are in large families: three or more adults plus one or more children. The differences are illustrated by Figure 3.

Figure 3 Types of families as a percentage of all households

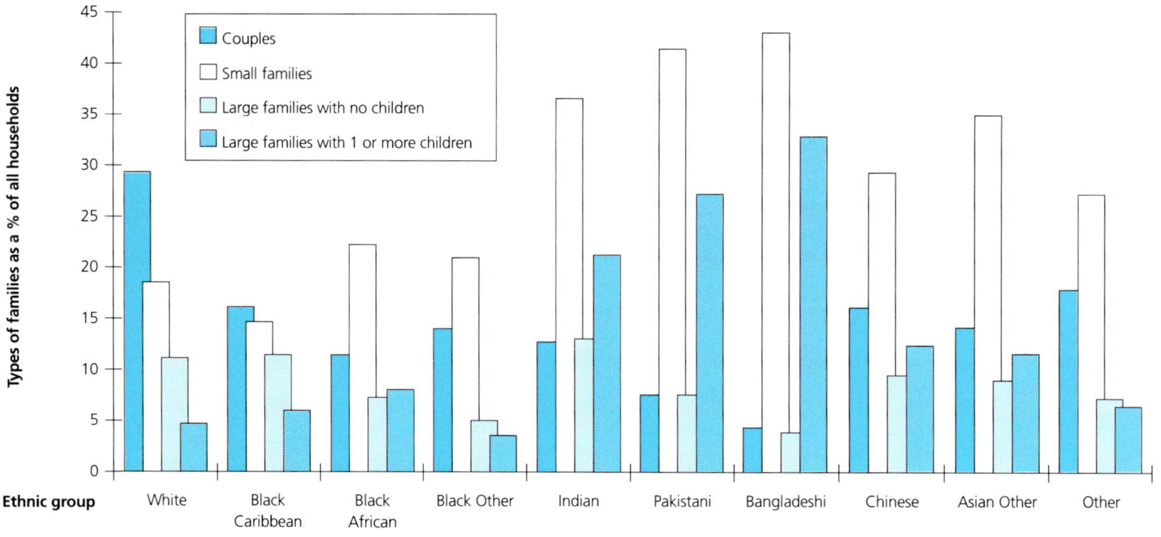

Source: Analysis presented by Owen. (1993c:4, Table 3)

Owen suggests that 'black' groups are similar to the 'white' ethnic group in that the number of households with dependent children are a minority (Owen, 1993c:13). However, it is unclear what impact the age profile of the different ethnic groups has: for example 'black' ethnic groups being comparatively older than other ethnic minority groups, therefore there may be more who are past their child-rearing years. In any case, Jones' analysis of the Labour Force Surveys for 1988/90 suggests that Afro-Caribbeans continue to have a slightly higher number of children under the age of 16 than is true for white households (Jones, 1993).

In overall terms Owen concludes that the nuclear family is by no means the most common type of household organisation. Families with children under the age of 16 were most common amongst Bangladeshis and Pakistanis, while single person households and childless couples are relatively uncommon in these groups. Owen contrasts this with black groups who tend to have higher proportions of lone single adult households, one parent families and households with adult members of the same gender (Owen, 1993c:13).

In presenting this evidence care must be taken in terms of what a snapshot survey can actually tell us about the significance of the make-up of families. There is a tendency to highlight what is normal or what is traditional regardless of the specificity in terms of time and space of particular forms of family formation: for example the British nuclear family is very much a result of a particular time and place. Furthermore, the Census uses a very particular measure of the 'family unit' (those people living under one roof) and this will tell us little about how care is organised and the networks families may or may not have to draw upon. Barn, for example, in her discussion of the methodology for her study notes the existence of children whose parents lived separately but had equal access (Barn, 1993:28).

In addition, migration patterns as well as existing settlement patterns of black communities suggest a positive (not just a negative) pull for black communities to remain in particular geographical areas. Flett and her colleagues have shown that once access to public housing became a possibility, black people continued to indicate their preference for accommodation in inner area wards even though these had comparatively the worst type of housing (Flett et al, 1979:290). As our discussion of 'spatial segregation' suggests, black communities continue to congregate in particular areas, even though these have high levels of social and economic deprivation.

With these caveats in mind, it is possible to conclude that for the majority of black communities, family units with children under the age of 16 are a common experience. Furthermore, these families are likely to have more children under the age of 16 then their white counterparts. Finally, the number of adults per family unit with children may vary from one to three or more, but the most common was two adults of different genders.

Child abuse and neglect

The 1989 Children Act has attempted to unify and give direction to the provision of the state's services to children and families. A central thrust in the Act is to impose a duty on local authorities to safeguard and promote the welfare of children in their area who are in need (Home Office, 1991:1). Clearly, the first step in that process is the investigation of abuse and neglect, yet as has been recently argued there is little research into how effectively those charged with these duties are protecting and promoting the welfare of black children (Phillips and Butt, 1996; Jones and Butt, 1995). Not surprisingly this is accompanied with little British research specifically examining the incidence or prevalence or characteristics of neglect and abuse within Britain's black communities.

An aspect of this latter failing is the almost inherent difficulty in exploring the incidence or prevalence of abuse, in particular sexual abuse. The Butler-Sloss report into child abuse in Cleveland specifically focused on the need to develop national estimates of incidence or prevalence of sexual abuse (Ghate and Spencer, 1995:1). However, as Ghate and Spencer (1995) suggest in their discussion of a feasibility study of a national survey of prevalence of child sexual abuse, this is far from straightforward. They further suggest there may be particular difficulties with people of different cultural backgrounds (Ghate and Spencer, 1995:41).

However, some evidence is beginning to appear. Gibbons et al (1995) in their examination of the operation of the child protection system do provide some comparative information in terms of three ethnic groups: 'white', 'black' and 'asian'. After noting the large amount of missing data on ethnic origin of the sample, Gibbons et al describe their findings:

> Black and asian families were over-represented among referrals for physical injury compared to whites (58% v 42%), and under-represented among referrals for sexual abuse (20% compared to 31%). Black african and asian families were more often referred for using an implement, such as a cane, to inflict physical injury: 40% of asians and 43% of black africans had beaten their children with a stick or other implement compared to 30% of afro-caribbeans and 16% of whites.

They continue:

> On the research measures, the consequences of the injuries inflicted on black and asian children were no more likely to be long-lasting: it was the form the punishment took that was unacceptable to community agents who referred these children. (Gibbons et al, 1995:40)

Some evidence from indirect sources does identify abuse or neglect. In a study exploring homelessness and running away from home, Patel suggests that while a number of people assumed that the reason young Asian women were running away was fear of arranged marriages, the reality was:

> Like many other young women in general, the young black women interviewed were running [away] because of physical violence, emotional and sexual abuse and other family conflicts. (Patel, 1994:35)

We may also conclude from the evidence of the higher risk of black communities experiencing poverty or deprivation (Robson et al, 1995:82 and 162) and its association with neglect and abuse (Gibbons et al, 1995:12) that we should find higher rates of abuse in black communities. However, Gibbons et al (1995) warn against relying on poverty as an indicator of the maltreatment of children, noting that their research suggests poverty does not wholly explain the variance in registration rates in different demographic areas. Furthermore Garbarino and Kostelny (1992), in summarising several American studies, suggest a much more complex relationship. While they note the association of socio-economic factors with abuse and neglect, they also suggest that where communities are more coherent, in that they have lower crime and violence rates, and a better sense of community, there tends to be a lower incidence of abuse. Whether this is true for Britain's black communities is difficult to say.

American studies - which appear to be of a larger scale - suggest that there is little variance between black and white communities' experiences of abuse and neglect. Finkelhor and Barron (1986) summarise the American evidence thus:

> Across the board, studies have consistently failed to find any black-white differences in rates of sexual abuse. Even among reported cases, in which it is thought that blacks suffer from a labelling bias . . ., the percentage of black cases is no more than the percentage of blacks in the population . . . (Finkelhor and Barron, 1986:69)

They continue:

> Among reported cases, sexual abuse has consistently been the type of abuse in which blacks have the lowest representation. In the American Humane Association National records . . . for example, black families accounted for 15.3% of sexual abuse cases, almost exactly their proportion in the American population. In the National Incidence Study . . . the percentage of blacks was 11%, somewhat below their representation in the population. This is especially significant considering that discrimination, poverty, and stereotyping usually influence professionals to more readily label black families as abusive. (Finkelhor and Barron, 1986:70)

Two possible conclusions emerge: the first is that there is evidence that black children, just as white children, are in need of protection to promote their welfare. While the evidence is limited, it nevertheless does suggest the existence of abuse and neglect. Second, the higher risk of black communities experiencing poverty and deprivation may suggest the possibility of higher rates of abuse or neglect. However, there is little evidence to support this, with the American literature suggesting there is little variance in abuse between black communities and their white counterparts, even though there may be a degree of discrimination in the relationship between professionals and black communities (see Butt, 1996 for a further discussion).

Black children in the care system

Barn, in her review of research on children in care, notes:

> Scant attention has been given to the situation of black children. To date, there has been no systematic research into the articulation and operationalisation of the statutory care of black children. (Barn, 1993:6)

While this may be overstating the case, the continuing failure of research on child in care to explore the experience of black children is certainly demonstrated by publications such as the Department of Health's Social Work Decisions in Child Care (1985). Of the nine studies summarised, none focuses on the experience of black children (Barn, 1993:7). The more recent examination of family support - Gibbons' The Children Act 1989 and Family Support (1992), another product summarising a series of DH funded research projects - does mention black children and families. However, those authors that do make a mention point to the limited coverage of black people by their research (for example Gibbons, 1992:4; or Smith, 1992:10).

Studies that have attempted to look at the number of black children in care, while not producing directly comparable information, have produced a similar picture. Foren and Batta (1970) suggested that Mixed Origin children are 8.5 times more likely to come into care than White Indigenous children as well as African Caribbean and Asian children (Foren and Batta, 1970:12). Batta et al repeated some of this work in their investigation of juvenile delinquency amongst Asian and Half Asians and came to a similar conclusion about the over-representation of Mixed Origin children in care (Batta at al, 1975). They further suggested that the number of Afro-Caribbean and Asian children coming into care had increased faster than for White children or children of Mixed Origin (Batta et al, 1975). As the 1980s began, Batta and Mawby returned to the investigation of children in care of Bradford Social Services and confirmed the earlier findings of over-representation of Mixed Origin children in care (Batta and Mawby, 1981:145).

A number of local authority based studies look at black children in care (Lambeth, 1981; Hackney, 1985; McAdam, 1987). In 1985 Hackney Social Services Department attempted to examine their own records to identify the ethnic composition of children in care. They found that of the 523 children in care 209 were either UK Black, Afro-Caribbean or African; 9 were Asian; and 231 were White. In similar fashion to Hackney, McAdam's study of children in care in Brent in 1986 does not identify whether black children are over-represented in care, but she does note their high numbers. She states that Afro-Caribbeans make up the largest single group: 171 girls and boys who account for 43 per cent of the 394 children in care (McAdam, 1987:29). Her unhappiness with the method of data collection does suggest we need to treat these figures with some care.

Barn's study, while considerably more complex than those referred to above, is once again a study of just one authority (which she calls Wenford): an empirical study which examines the care careers of black children in an inner city local authority social services department. The research was based on a combination of qualitative and quantitative methods which included a precoded questionnaire for a documentary analysis of case files and reports, together with interviews with social workers and parents (both natural and foster). In total 564 children participated in the study: 294 were black and 270 white. Barn summarises her findings thus:

> By comparing 'in care' age groups to the child population figures the Wenford research was able to establish that black children were over-represented in care, and that the majority of the cohort group were under the age of five when they entered care. The situation for Mixed Origin children did not differ significantly from those of African Caribbean origin (Barn, 1993:50)

Rowe et al, who admit that they had not considered all the ramifications of their interest in ethnic origin in their study of the placement of children, provide additional support for the over-representation of black children in 'admissions' to care. They note:

> that black children were over-represented in admissions to care of all six project authorities, although the extent to which this was happening varied. (Rowe et al, 1989:163)

They proceed to suggest, however, that much of this can be accounted for by the large number of young black children being admitted for temporary care during family emergencies and leaving care soon afterward.

In 1987 Bebbington and Miles carried out a survey of 13 of the 108 local authorities in England. The family background of all children formally taken into care was monitored for a period of six months. They found that:

> Single-race children from ethnic minorities are not over-represented amongst the children entering care, especially when

allowance is made for other factors from the samples. Afro-Caribbean and African children are a little more likely to come into care than white children, but the differences are not statistically significant. On the other hand, a child of mixed race is two-and-a-half times as likely to enter care as a white child, all else being equal. (Bebbington and Miles, 1989:356)

The failure of the Bebbington and Miles, the Rowe et al and the Barn studies to show a consistent picture across the board has been commented on already. Why this is so can be speculated upon. First, their analysis is based on differing cohorts: the Rowe et al sample is based on all children admitted to care whereas Barn's sample is drawn from children in care. Therefore it is no surprise that Rowe et al note the large number of black children admitted temporarily during family crisis as this is a feature of those admitted to care as opposed to those in care (Timæus, 1990:379). Second, they have approached the question of the representation of black children in care from a different starting point. While Barn specifically sets out to explore the experience of black children, for the other two studies it is but one element of the research. This is demonstrated in both the Rowe et al and Bebbington and Miles sampling techniques: whereas they expend considerable effort in attempting to gain a range of representative authorities, they do not consider whether their authorities are representative of the experience of black communities. Rowe et al admit that while some comparison of their data with that of Batta and Mawby is possible, they do not have a Bradford equivalent in their sample (Rowe et al, 1989:159).

Third, it may also be a result of the differing ways that the information was collected and how successful each was in their endeavours: Rowe et al required social workers to provide all the information historical and current; Bebbington and Miles again required social workers to provide all the information but for new cases only and suffered lower than expected returns for two authorities; Barn collected all the information herself through an examination of case records. Finally, while Rowe et al and Bebbington and Miles attach considerable importance to the disaggregated ethnic minority group categories there is little discussion as to why they use particular categories (none in the case of Bebbington and Miles). The Bebbington and Miles omission is particularly puzzling, because while they make references to Africans this group is not presented in the published tables. Conversely Barn, who puts least emphasis on the disaggregated ethnic minority groupings, discusses them at greatest length. We could speculate that if all three studies chose to present their analysis in an aggregated form there might be less variation in their conclusions.

Recognising these limitations, it is possible to argue that there is some consistency. The local studies do show significant representation of black children (particularly those of Caribbean origin) in care and those that explore this issue show over-representation. Furthermore, Rowe et al's study gives some support to this. Most of the studies suggest children with one white and one black parent may also be over-represented: Bebbington and Miles suggest that they are two-and-a-half times as likely as a white child to enter care.

When the figures on black children in care are disaggregated another consistent picture emerges. While as noted Batta and his colleagues' work identifies over-representation of Asian children in care, other studies (Rowe et al, 1989:163; Barn, 1993:21 and 33) highlight their under-representation or that their numbers were no higher than might be expected (Bebbington and Miles, 1989:355 and 356). This picture is confirmed by other local studies, for example McAdam (1987). Whether the 'lower' number of Asian children is reflective of some studies not covering departments with sizeable Asian populations is unclear, but the low number of Asian children is a salient feature.

All the studies referred to above had their data collection phase around or before 1987, a full two years before the Children Act reached the statute book and four years before it was implemented (October 1991). Additionally, none of these studies is able to reflect on change over time, except for Batta et al (1981) who are able to do so in only a limited way. A more recent picture, that also provides evidence for change over two years, can be drawn from Nottinghamshire County Council's annual statistical reports on children's services (NCC, n.d.). The number of black children in care on 31st March 1990 and 1991 is presented in Table 7.

The authors conclude that the number of black children in care has increased to almost 1 in every 10. They further state in terms of those admitted to care there had been 148 admissions in the year 1990/91:

> Numerically, admissions involving black children increased over the previous year by 19% (the 1989/90 figure was 124); this compares with the 3% overall decrease in admissions. As a result, the proportion of admissions involving black children rose from 12% to 15%. (NCC, n.d.:6)

Importantly, it appears that while Nottinghamshire is following the national trend in decline in admissions (Timæus, 1990:377), the same may not be true for black children.

Table 7   Ethnic origin of children in care as at 31st March 1990 and 1991

Ethnic group	31 March 90 n	31 March 90 %	31 March 91 n	31 March 91 %
Afro-Caribbean	62	3.1	51	2.5
African	2	0.1	2	0.1
Indian	2	0.1	4	0.2
Pakistani	8	0.4	13	0.6
Other Asian	2	0.1	2	0.1
Mixed - Afro-Caribbean/White	67	3.3	92	4.5
Mixed - Asian/White	18	0.9	17	0.8
Mixed - Other	16	0.8	15	0.7
White	1833	91.1	1857	90.2
Other	2	0.1	6	0.3
Black	179	8.9	202	9.8
White	1833	91.1	1857	90.2

Source: Nottinghamshire County Council

Age and gender

While the debate on over and under-representation has dominated research on black children in care, more recent research has begun to explore some of the characteristics of these children and their 'care careers', and this section will summarise the main findings. Barn, after noting that 58 per cent of black children were under five years old on entry into care, suggests that in her cohort there is no significant difference between white and black children with regard to age upon entry into care (Barn, 1993:165). The Nottinghamshire study suggests that in 1990/91, 1 in 4 admissions of under fives was black (NCC, n.d.:7). Rowe et al suggest that the number of pre-school admissions is high for all their six authorities. However they go on to show that it is an even more prominent feature of black admissions, and when considering admissions of mixed parentage children about half were under five (Rowe et al, 1989:165).

Rowe et al suggest that an explanation of their findings regarding age is that a large number of black children had been admitted as a temporary measure after a family emergency, with 58 per cent of Afro-Caribbeans, 66 per cent of African and 62 per cent of Asian expected to return home. Barn does not provide a similar analysis but does argue that while there is no significant difference in terms of ages of children in care at the time of entry, there is certainly evidence of over-representation in terms of age when compared to the child population of Wenford: the proportion of black children in care was higher than that in the child population for under fives; for 5 to 15 year olds; and possibly for 16 to 18 year olds (Barn, 1993:48).

Few studies provide information on the gender make-up of black children in care even though this appears to influence some aspects of the care careers of black children: for example Knapp et al suggest that black boys are less likely to be fostered than white boys (Knapp et al, 1988). Barn however does look at her sample in terms of gender and suggests that while African Caribbean boys and girls are equally represented, the number of girls of Mixed Origin is higher than boys. She further concludes:

> It is clear that white girls have a much lower chance of being admitted into care than black girls (African Caribbean and Mixed Origin). (Barn, 1993:46)

Family background

Commentaries suggest (Bebbington and Miles, 1989) that a sizeable literature exists on the family characteristics of children who have entered local authority care. The picture for black children is more complex. While many of the pre-1980 studies of black children in care provide information on the characteristics of their families (usually as an explanation of why these children were in care), the 1980s itself has seen a dearth of such information. This is probably a result of a move in research on black communities away from focusing on the communities to their experience of British society (Bourne, 1981). However the characteristics of families continues to play a part in research on children in care: Bebbington and Miles have used their 'children entering care survey' to develop a 'formula' from which they claim it is:

> possible to predict the probability that a child will enter care during the course of a year, given both their characteristics and the circumstances of their families. (Bebbington and Miles 1989:354)

They proceed to illustrate the probabilities for two children: see Figure 4

We have already questioned the definitions that Bebbington and Miles have used in terms of ethnicity, and their willingness to use different terms to describe the same type of household - 'broken families', 'single adult household', 'single parent family' - gives more cause for concern with regard to their analysis. Furthermore, their predictors seem to suggest little influence from the state, the operation of (discriminatory) practice and certainly none from self-fulfilling prophecy, which often suggests that if certain types of families are seen as dysfunctional, it is likely that these are the ones who will be investigated. However, our interest here is that once again we see the family circumstances of those in care being focused upon.

Figure 4 Bebbington and Miles' illustration of the probability of entering care

Child A	Child B
Aged 5 to 9	Aged 5 to 9
No supplementary benefit	Household head receives
Two parent family	supplementary benefit
Three or fewer children	Single adult household
White	Four or more children
Owner occupied home	Mixed ethnic origin
More rooms than people	Private rented home
	One or more persons per room
Odds are 1 in 7,000	*Odds are 1 in 10*

Source: Bebbington and Miles (1989:354)

The information available from all the studies on the family circumstances of these children is minimal. Bebbington and Miles have some of this information, but do not disaggregate for black children, while Rowe et al do not ask for it, nor do many of the local studies. However, Barn notes that 83 per cent of the black children in care came from single parent families, most of which were mother-headed units. Importantly, black children were much more likely to be from higher socio-economic groups, with 47 per cent of black children's mothers coming from white collar or skilled manual occupations (Barn, 1993:101). Barn concludes from this that we must be careful not to forward the usual deprivation explanations when trying to understand black children's experience of social care (Barn, 1993:104).

Legal status
In terms of legal status on entry into care Barn and Rowe et al present a very similar picture. As these studies pre-date the 1989 Children Act, there were essentially two routes of entry under Section 2 of the 1980 Children Act, described by all those studied as the voluntary route and the compulsory route, which essentially drew on the 1969 Children and Young Persons Act. Barn notes the statistically significant relationship between the number of black children entering care and their more likely use of the 'voluntary route'. While Rowe et al show a higher rate of voluntary admission for white children in comparison to Barn's study, they still identify its dominance as the route of entry for black children (Rowe at al, 1989:168): see Figure 5.

Turning to the compulsory route, Rowe and her colleagues note:

Figure 5 Percentage of voluntary admissions by ethnic group and age

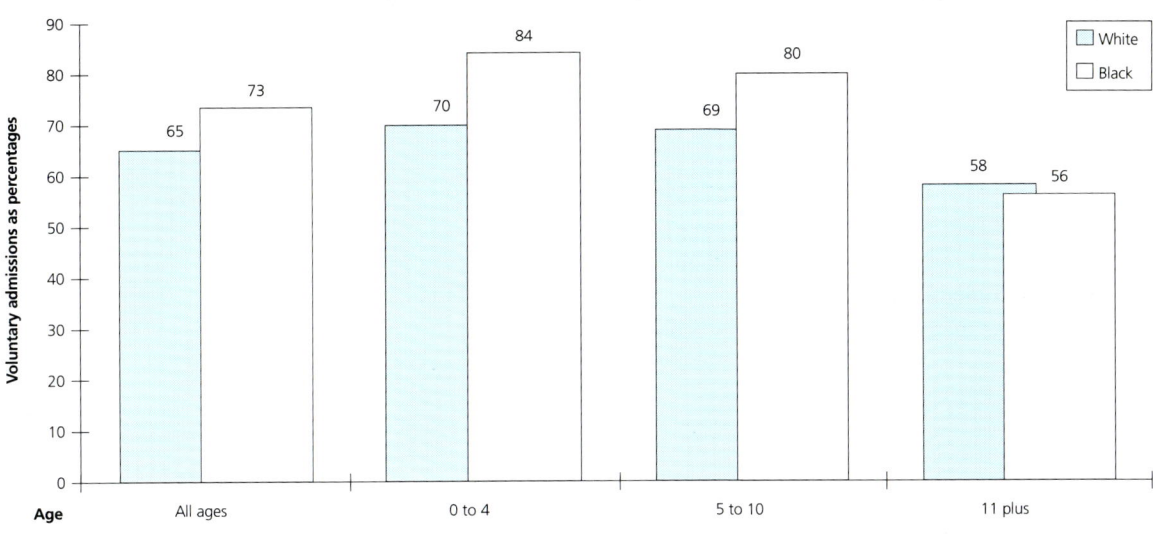

Source: Rowe et al (1989:169)

In comparison to whites, only about half as many young black children were admitted on place of safety orders. Mixed parentage children of all ages were the most likely to be on care orders through care proceedings. By contrast not one Asian child or young person was admitted on a care order. (Rowe et al, 1989:169)

Barn suggests that for her cohort the situation changes quickly after a period in care from dominance of the voluntary entry to compulsory. She summarised the changes thus:

- from voluntary care to the assumption of parental rights and duties by the local authority

- from a place of safety order/interim care order . . . to a full care order

- from voluntary care to wardship. (Barn, 1993:44)

To summarise, all the studies show that the majority of black children in care or admitted to care were under the age of five on entry. There was little evidence of significant numbers of black teenagers entering care, although Barn notes that when compared with the child population of the local authority she investigated, black 16 to 18 year olds were probably over-represented. Barn's is the only study that explores gender differences, noting that black girls were more likely than white girls to be admitted to care. In terms of family circumstances, Barn provides the greatest amount of detail, noting

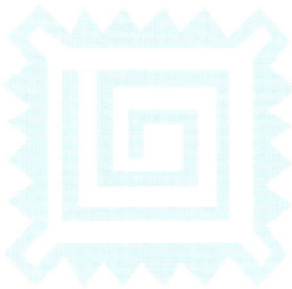

the dominance of female lone parent households with a significant
number of women in white collar and skilled manual occupations.

All the work that examines legal status notes black children's entry
into care through the voluntary route (Section 2 of the 1980
Children Act), and this was significantly so in comparison to white
children. However, Barn suggests that within a short period of being
in care black children were likely to experience a change in their
legal status, which would see them move from voluntary to
compulsory status: in effect becoming more like their white
counterparts.

The placement of children

As we have noted, in addition to the debate around the number of
black children in care there has been considerable controversy about
the family placement of children who have been in care (Rhodes,
1992:1). While the research that has not set out to look at black
children specifically has been dominated by various debates, including
the relative merits of fostering as opposed to adoption, the research
in terms of black children specifically has almost exclusively focused
on the transracial placement of black children. It is important to note
that the debate is entirely about the transracial placement of black
children and those with one black and one white parent, not about
white children. As Cheetham notes, social workers were always reluctant to place a white child with a black family even when white
families were not available and black families were (Cheetham, 1981),
and none of the studies consulted here identifies a single placement
of a white child with a black family.

Gill and Jackson's study of transracially placed children ignited the
controversy in this country with their claims that transracial
placement had little impact on the self-esteem of these children.
However, some of these issues had been explored in America by
Horowitz in 1936 and Clark and Clark in 1939 (Banks, 1992:19),
amongst a number of other more recent interventions (Shaw,
1988:91). The consequence of this controversy is that considerable
effort has been spent on exploring notions of self-esteem or self-con-
cept or racial identity (Tizard and Phoenix, 1989; Biehal et al, 1995)
However little attention has been paid to other measures of the
'success' of the family placement of children such as breakdown of
placements or length of placements, or placements achieving what
they were set out to do: all factors which have been prominent in the
'mainstream' research (Triseliotis, 1989:6). Clearly identity is a
particular issue for those who have been adopted or fostered (Walby
and Symons, 1990; Banks, 1992), but much of the debate has been
polemical rather than illuminating. Our discussion, rather than re-vis-

iting this ground, will try and explore some of the other findings of research on the placement of black children.

Fratter and her colleagues (1991) have documented the rise of the 'permanence movement' which increasingly saw the permanent placement of children in adoptive families as the best form of care for children who were in care. This was not only the result of unhappiness with fostering and residential child care, but was a product of changes such as the decline in the number of healthy babies, which was accompanied by a growth in interest in the adoption of:

> older children, those with difficulties, and black and mixed parentage children. These previously had been considered almost unpalatable . . . (Fratter et al, 1991:10)

They further recount that these were the changes that were behind Rowe and Lambert's study Children Who Wait? (1973), which first explored the assertions by potential adoptive parents that while they waited to adopt there were children 'languishing in care'. Rowe and Lambert concluded that there were indeed a number of children who were no longer in contact with their birth families and required substitute families. In terms of black children they found that of the 2760 children in their survey, 552 were black. Around 388 of them were 'confined' to residential care but there were 164 who could be adopted (Rowe and Lambert, 1973).

The fact that one in five of these children in residential establishments was black appeared to concur with other studies and leads Barn to conclude that 'the overwhelming finding has been that black children are over-represented in residential establishments' (Barn, 1993:69).

There is some evidence to suggest that while Barn is correct, her conclusion is true only for the 1970s (all except one of the studies she quotes are from the 1970s). McAdam's study of Brent suggests that for the majority of children 'boarding out' (placement in a foster home) was the most likely placement: 68 per cent of Afro-Caribbean children; 65 per cent of Asian children; and 69 per cent of white children. The Hackney study notes that of 523 children, 239 were in foster homes and implies little difference in the rates of fostering between black and white groups. Whilst the Nottinghamshire study does not identify placements by ethnic origin, it too suggests that 'boarding out' is the most popular placement. Furthermore, Rowe et al suggest that for their sample:

> Rather surprisingly, in view of concern about finding foster homes for black children, we found that fostering rates for

white, Afro-Caribbean and mixed parentage children were almost identical. The proportion of Asian children fostered appears lower . . . (Rowe et al, 1989:170)

Barn notes a further caveat and that is a lower number of black children were allowed 'home on trial', a point supported by Rowe et al (1989).

Barn's own study suggests that black children (51 per cent) had a much better chance of being placed in a substitute family than white children (38 per cent). However when considering black children only, they were as likely to be placed in a substitute family as residential accommodation (Barn, 1993:61).

To summarise, even with some evidence of the continued presence of black children in residential establishments it is clear that family placement is becoming the dominant form of care for black children, as it appears to be for most children (Berridge and Cleaver, 1987:3).

Outcomes

As social work begins to assess the impact of its interventions we are beginning to see emerge evidence on outcomes for children in care. However, the possibility of comparing the various studies that do have information on outcomes for black children in care[6] (Berridge and Cleaver, 1987; Rowe et al, 1989; Bebbington and Miles 1989; Fratter et al, 1991; Charles et al, 1992; Barn, 1993; Biehal et al, 1995) is particularly problematic. Firstly they draw on different cohorts of black children in care; secondly they use significantly different measures; finally some do not draw any information from the children themselves or their birth families, or their new families. The approach we adopt is therefore to briefly present the findings of each study, and then draw some speculative conclusions.

Berridge and Cleaver (1987) examined the incidence and causes of foster home breakdown for 372 children. After warning about the possible bias in their data set, they report as far as long term foster care is concerned:

> From our evidence and using our definition of outcome, we would not conclude that the association between the racial characteristics of foster parents and children is paramount, although there was some tendency for mixed race children placed with white, long term foster parents to experience more breakdowns than one might expect.

After highlighting the success of some agencies in recruiting black foster parents for intermediate foster placements, they note:

Of the 20 intermediate placements involving black children (14 of whom were located with black families), only 2 (ten per cent) ended prematurely. (Berridge and Cleaver, 1987:67)

They further note of the 32 mixed race children 27 were placed with white families and the breakdown rate was a 'low' per cent. The breakdown rate for white children in white families was 27 per cent (p137). This evidence leads Triseliotis to speculate that black children placed with black families may be experiencing better outcomes than white children placed with white families (Triseliotis, 1989).

Rowe at al (1989), who define success rates as achieving what was planned on admission to care, note that they 'can say with considerable confidence that, in many respects, outcomes for black children and white children are essentially similar' (p174). However, they too identify some differences:

Looking across all types of placement, we find that slightly more black teenagers had 'successful' endings (45 per cent compared to 24 per cent white). Within the black group, Asian and mixed parentage teenagers had somewhat higher proportion of 'successful' placements than did Afro-Caribbeans and Africans. When foster home and residential endings are compared, Afro-Caribbeans seem to have had high 'success' ratings for foster home endings and low ones for residential endings, whereas for Asians the pattern was reversed. (Rowe et al, 1989:174)

Barn (1993) explores rehabilitation and discharge and notes that:

Level of contact between natural parents and children is a cru-cial contributory factor, leading to the rehabilitation and discharge of children from care. The Wenford study showed that a greater proportion of black children than white children had regular contact with their parents . . . Where there was no con-tact at all, the majority of children and families were white.(Barn, 1993:91)

She adds:

It was found that the very reason for black children's greater contact with their parents was the fact that they were placed in black foster families. Black children in transracial families did not experience the same degree of regular contact as those in same race placements. (Barn, 1993:100)

Finally, she states:

The route of exit for the majority of these children was withdrawal from voluntary care. (Barn, 1993:100)

Fratter et al (1991), who carried out a survey of 1165 children with 'special needs' placed by major voluntary agencies with permanent new families between 1984 and 1987, examined success in terms of those still living with their new family, or in continued contact (p28) and disruption (irrevocable breakdown). Fratter et al suggest that 29 per cent of mixed parentage children experienced disrupted placements (a statistically significant difference p < .05) as did 27 per cent of the black children (not significant). The breakdown rate for the white children was 20 per cent and that for a small number in the 'other' category 12 per cent. The statistical evidence suggests that neither having two black nor two white parents is significantly associated with outcome, but being of mixed parentage is a risk factor in that it is associated with negative outcomes. (Fratter et al, 1991:40)

Charles at al (1992) have explored the same group of children as the above study, but have added 37 children under the age of three to the sample, as well as collecting information on the characteristics of the new families children were placed with. They note:

> When risk or protective factors are held constant . . . the multivariate analysis indicates that children both of whose parents are black are neither more nor less likely to experience breakdown than white children, but that black children of mixed parentage are more likely to experience breakdown. (Charles et al, 1992:18)

After noting the small numbers in their sample does not allow further multivariate analysis (controlling for various risk factors) to be carried out, they speculate that if this was possible it would show little difference in breakdown rates between black children placed with black families and white children placed with white families. However:

> There would be a tendency for the children placed transracially to be more likely to experience breakdown. (Charles et al, 1992:18)

The variability in measuring outcome, amongst a range of other inconsistencies, makes it a particularly arduous task to draw any conclusions from these studies regarding outcome or to attach too much weight to them. However, there is some suggestion that black children placed with black families will share similar (or better) outcomes to white children placed with white families. Furthermore, black children appear to benefit from the 'protective' factor of continued contact with their birth families and black foster and adoptive parents may be particularly able in managing this. However, children with one black and one white parent appear to be particularly at risk of unsuccessful outcomes and are less likely to have the protection of continued contact with their birth family.

Conclusion

There can be little doubt that black children need to be protected, just as white children do. Similarly they need to have their welfare promoted. While the development of preventative strategies seems to be indicated by the significant number of black children entering care on a voluntary basis, the evidence appears to suggest a lack of access to and use of these services (Smith, 1989). The opposite appears to be the case in terms of accessing compulsory care. For children who have one black parent and one white there is little disagreement about their over-representation. For children whose parents are both black the national studies appear to be in disagreement with the local studies. The national studies suggest that where there is over-representation this disappears when controlling for age. However the local studies do show over-representations of black children.

The placement of black children once in care remains controversial. Fratter et al (1991) recount the changes in the placement of black children from being deemed unplaceable, to being placed almost exclusively with white families at the beginning of the 1980s, to the majority (but not all) being placed with black families by the end of that decade. There is some evidence that black children have better outcomes with black families and that black foster carers are more readily able to manage the greater likelihood of black children maintaining contact with their birth family. There is also evidence that children with one parent black and one parent white are more likely to experience breakdown. How much this is due to their regular placement with white families is unclear.

The research evidence considered here, while showing some patterns, continues to be problematic. We are beginning to see studies that build on existing work, either continuing work such as in the case of Charles et al, or assessing existing studies such as in that of Barn. However, much of the work considered here uses different starting points, categorises ethnicity in different ways, uses different methods of investigation and considers various methods of assessing outcomes. Additionally, certain areas remain unexplored: we can draw little evidence about family support or preventative work with black children and their families, for instance. The importance of gender or disability is rarely investigated.

From our earlier discussion of the incidence and prevalence of abuse or neglect in black communities, it is likely that the evidence discussed in the rest of this chapter is an indication of agencies attempting to respond to the social care needs of black children and their families. However, this chapter also suggests that there is much more work to be done before we can assess if any of this work has helped to protect or promote the welfare of black children.

4

Black elders

Summary

The extensive research on black elders does not hide the fact that there are several gaps, including few national studies, but the quantity of research does allow us to build a reasonably sound picture. Black pensioners are comparatively younger than their white counterparts. However their 'youth' does not appear to protect them from frailty and illness. A number of studies show levels of ill health and difficulties in performing basic tasks normally associated with older people in England.

These greater levels of frailty and ill-health are accompanied by comparatively worse economic and housing conditions. A greater proportion of black elders derive some or all of their income from means tested welfare benefits at the same time as a smaller number receiving occupational or full state pensions. In addition, while significant numbers of black elders are owner-occupiers they still constitute a smaller proportion than their white counterparts. Of greater significance is that they own the worst type of accommodation, often without the benefit of basic amenities.

The stereotype of black elders living in multi-generational households appears to still hold true. However a salient feature of these studies is the challenge they pose to the ability of these 'extended' families to cater for the needs of black older people: often it appears not to be a case of care, but of containment.

Sadly the studies also suggest that at present social care agencies (whether from social services or from health) are not in a position to meet the social care needs of black elders. There are various barriers ranging from lack of knowledge of services, to racism, or to inappropriate services.

Importantly for social care providers the 1980s has seen a dramatic rise in this group of older people: 168 per cent between 1981 and 1991. While the actual numbers appear less dramatic, the growth illustrates the need for service providers to put appropriate service provision to black communities on their agenda.

The research on black elders is remarkable because of the sheer quantity of material in comparison to other areas of social care and black communities. However much of the research discussed here is the result of small scale local studies. Most often the funders, as well as those carrying out the work, were concerned with the policy and practice implications for service development rather than the incidence and prevalence of needs. Therefore the reports spend more space discussing how needs should be met rather than what these needs are. This inevitably impacts on our review, requiring some attention to be paid to access and delivery.

In this context it is also important to note a salient feature of the majority of large scale national studies: they have universally failed to focus on black elders. When discussing samples these studies rarely detail whether any black people are part of the sample; in describing findings they rarely note whether the experience of black elders is different or the same; and in drawing conclusions they do not state whether they are true for black elders or not.

Double jeopardy and triple jeopardy

Before reviewing the relevant studies, we need to deal with the concepts of double and triple jeopardy which have become an integral part of the debate on black elders' experience of care.

The notion of 'double jeopardy' has arisen out of a growing concern in American literature on the relationship between ethnicity and ageing (Williams [1990] has summarised the American literature on double jeopardy - Driedger and Chappell, 1987; Gelfand and Kutzick, 1979; Holzberg, 1982). For example, she notes that the American literature defines the concept of 'double jeopardy' in relation to black older people to mean the suffering of cumulative disadvantages due to racial discrimination (or to discrimination against their ethnic culture) as well as the risks associated with old age (Williams, 1990:109).

In Britain, this has been taken up and extended to one of 'triple jeopardy' (Norman, 1985). 'Triple jeopardy' attempts to add to the concept of 'double jeopardy' the concern that black older people's needs are not being met by the present health and social services systems. Norman (1985) summarises thus:

> They are not merely in double jeopardy by reason of age and discrimination, as has often been stated, but in triple jeopardy, at risk because they are old, because of the physical conditions and hostility under which they have to live, and because services are not accessible to them. (Norman, 1985:1)

While the concept of triple jeopardy is useful because it focuses on the various sources of discrimination in the lives of black elderly people, it is problematic. Triple jeopardy conveys a notion of distinct and separate forms of discrimination (age and race) that can be added together in some form of mathematical sum (see Begum, 1994). The reality, however, is that black elderly people experience discrimination in ways that rarely differentiate between age or race, in similar fashion to the experience of black disabled people (see chapter 6).

Demography

A feature of the presence of black communities in Great Britain has been their relative 'youth' in comparison to white people (see chapter 2, page 19). For example, the overall median age of white people is 37.4 but for black groups it is 25.5: a difference of over 12 years (Owen, 1993a). However there is evidence of a rapidly growing number of black elderly people.

During 1984-6 about 2.43 million (4.5 per cent) of the total population in Britain were from black and minority ethnic communities (Labour Force Survey, 1984/1986). Of these around 97,280 persons were over 60. These included about 38,000 persons of Indian origin, 32,000 of either West Indian or Guyanese origin, 7,940 of Pakistani origin, 1,030 of Bangladeshi origin and 5,750 of Chinese origin. The data did not illuminate gender differences, but according to Fenton (1987) because of the differences in migration patterns 'men will outnumber women among black older people'. However, more recent evidence from the 1991 Census suggests equal numbers of male and female black older people rather than more men or more women (see chapter 2, page 20).

According to the 1991 Census 15.18 per cent of the total population from black communities were aged between 45-64 years and 3.22 per cent were post retirement age (aged 60 for women and 65 for men). For the white community the corresponding figures were 22.32 per cent aged between 45-64 years and 16.80 per cent post retirement age. Of the total population in Great Britain black people aged between 45-64 years account for 3.80 per cent and 1.10 per cent of those aged 65 plus. Though the proportion of black older people compared to white older people is small, it is clear that it has been and is growing. For example, Owen (1993a) details the changes between 1981 and 1991 of various age cohorts and suggests that while the number of New Commonwealth and Pakistan people who are between 45 and pensionable age has grown by 35 per cent, the largest percentage growth has been in those people of pensionable age: 168.6 per cent (from 61,200 in 1981 to 164,306 in 1991).

Spatial location

We have already noted that black communities are clustered in
certain parts of England. While there is some evidence that black
communities are moving from their traditional areas into the suburbs,
this may not be true for black elderly people who appear to be still
living in inner city wards.

Limiting long term illness

For the first time the 1991 Census included a question on limiting
long term illness. Though its usefulness is limited by the fact that it
treats all types of health problems as being of equal severity, some
researchers have used it as an indicator of the general level of health
of the population. The 1991 Census recorded that the total number
of residents in a household in Great Britain that had a long term limiting illness was 6.67 million: 12.4 per cent of the total population.
The proportion with limiting long term illness increased with age.
For example, amongst those between pensionable age and 74 years
old, 30.2 per cent had a long term limiting illness. For those aged
between 75-84 years old the figure was 45.7 per cent and for those
aged 85 and over the figure was 62.2 per cent. Among the black
communities the proportion of the population with limiting long
term illness ranged from a 'low' of 4.4 per cent for the Chinese to
11.2 per cent among the Black Caribbean group (Charlton et al,
1994). Again, as in the white population, the incidence of limiting
long term illness increased with age (see chapter 6, page 88). When
standardised for age, Charlton et al (1994) found that rates of limiting long term illness were lowest for Chinese men and women, and
highest for Bangladeshi men and Pakistani women. In general
women's rates tended to be higher than those for men, except for
white, Bangladeshi and Chinese groups.

Household composition

Households with pensioners in the white communities account for
almost 26 per cent (around 5393.6 thousand households) of all white
households, while for black communities they account for just over 4
per cent (around 36.3 thousand households). Of the ethnic minority
groups, the largest number of households with pensioners are Black
Caribbeans with 7.2 per cent (around 15.5 thousand households), followed by the Chinese with 3.7 per cent (around 2 thousand households) and Indians with 3.6 per cent (just over 8 thousand
households). The proportion of lone pensioner households within
the black communities was 2.8 per cent (around 24.7 thousand households) compared to 15.6 per cent (around 3277.6 thousand households) for the white community. Again, Black Caribbeans had a
higher proportion compared to all other minority ethnic groups with
5.3 per cent (around 11.6 thousand households), followed by 2.4 per

cent (around 1.2 thousand households) for the Chinese and 2 per cent (around 4.4 thousand households) for Indians (see chapter 2, page 22).

Health and social care needs

Studies conducted over the last 15 years have explored the health and social care needs of black older people living in Britain (Farrah, 1986; Donaldson and Odell, 1984; Barker, 1984; Berry et al, 1981; Fenton, 1987; Turnbull, 1985; Bhalla and Blakemore, 1981; Lee, 1987). An emerging theme amongst all is that, though the sample of black older people was relatively young compared to white older people, considerable health and social care needs were discovered. For example, Farrah (1986) found that though two thirds of his sample (70 people out of 109) was only aged between 55 years and 69 years, 89 per cent of the sample studied reported poor eyesight, 12 per cent reported hearing difficulties, 28 per cent dental problems, 30 per cent feet and walking difficulties, 22 per cent were suffering from diabetes, 39 per cent from high blood pressure and 51 per cent from arthritis. Over a third (34 per cent) of those who reported health problems also said that their activities were restricted because of ill health, in particular mobility. In addition to the health problems, a higher proportion than expected for the age group also reported difficulties with self care and domestic tasks. Farrah found that 25 per cent had difficulty getting in and out of the bath and 11 per cent had difficulty getting to and using the toilet.

Donaldson and Odell (1984) noted similar problems for the Asian older people participating in their study. For example, 16 per cent of those aged 65-69 reported difficulty with going out of doors, 14 per cent reported difficulty with mobility within the home, 31 per cent reported difficulty climbing stairs, 8 per cent reported difficulty dressing themselves, 11 per cent reported difficulty bathing by themselves, and 12 per cent reported occasional and frequent incontinence. In addition between 8 per cent and 23 per cent reported difficulty with undertaking household tasks unaided such as cooking, shopping, washing dishes, washing clothes, ironing, making beds and cleaning. The study also found that the proportion of people able to perform the above activities fell with increasing age. For example, 59 per cent of those aged 75 and over had difficulty going out of doors alone and of these 19 per cent would need someone's help.

Berry et al (1981) in a study of Afro-Caribbean older people in Nottingham reported varying degrees of mobility and health problems. For example, 18 per cent (26 people) of the sample reported difficulty getting about the house and 55 per cent (81 people) reported a recent illness. The most commonly reported problems were hypertension, arthritis/rheumatism, diabetes and strokes/paralysis. More women reported illnesses or disabilities than men. Respondents also reported difficulty with self care and domestic tasks (see Table 8). Almost 45 per cent of the sample (66 people out of 148 people) was aged between 60 years and 64 years and 15 per cent of the sample (22 people) was under age 60 years old.

Table 8 Illnesses or disabilities reported by respondents by gender

	Male	Female
Arthritis, Rheumatism	6	15
Cardiac conditions	2	2
Pulmonary conditions	0	1
Effects of accidents	7	4
Hypertension	8	25
Gastric/Intestinal complaints	4	1
Strokes, Paralysis	6	5
Diabetes	2	12
Nervous conditions	2	2
Other specific illnesses	1	6
Old age, vague answers	0	2
Total reported illnesses	38	75
Number of people interviewed	68	80

Source: Berry et al (1981).

Black older people and general practitioners

In contrast to community health and social services, many of the studies reviewed suggest a greater use of GPs by black older people than is the case for white people. Bhalla and Blakemore (1981) found that a greater proportion of both Asians and Afro-Caribbeans had visited their GP in the last month compared to white Europeans (68 per cent and 70 per cent respectively compared to 57 per cent). Fenton (1987) found that a higher proportion of black older people visited their GPs compared to white older people. For example, 66 per cent of the over 60s reported a problem requiring regular GP visits, as did 50 per cent of the 45-59 year old group. Fenton notes that:

> It is likely that much ill health is related to working lives. Many respondents spoke about accidents at work and the effect on their health of many years of arduous employment including unhealthy foundry work, building work and amongst women nursing and hospital domestic work (Fenton, 1987:28).

Balarajan et al (1989) found significant differences between ethnic groups in the rate of GP consultations: Afro-Caribbean and Indian men were the highest consulters. McCormick et al (1990) in their national study of general practice morbidity showed that men from the Indian subcontinent were generally more likely to consult general practitioners than those of UK origin, particularly for serious illness.

The Health and Lifestyles survey by the Health Education Authority (1994) shows that for both Asian older men and women (aged between 50 and 74 years), the number of visits to the GP within a year is higher than the average. For the UK population the average was 5.6 for women and 5.4 for men (Table 31, p 58). But for Asian women the number of consultation was between 9 and 12 in a year, whilst for men it was between 8.5 and 15 consultations. For Afro-Caribbean women the number of consultations in a year was the same as the UK average, whilst for Afro-Caribbean older men the number of consultations was slightly higher: 6.1 consultations.

The reasons for high consulting rates amongst black older people has not been systematically explored (Pharoah, 1995). For this reason care must be taken not to assume that higher rates of consulting necessarily mean greater frailty or illness amongst black older people but it certainly appears to lend support to this contention: particularly in light of the evidence on the prevalence of limiting illness or disability, which suggests on average a higher proportion of limiting illness or disability amongst the 'non-white' population (42.8 per cent compared to 27 per cent) for those aged between 50 and 74 years of age (Health Education Authority, 1994).

To summarise, it is possible on the basis of these studies to argue that black people do have social care needs and these emerge at a younger age than for their white counterparts. Further, although the 1991 Census evidence suggests little difference in the prevalence of long-term limiting illness, it is likely that a more detailed examination would show higher rates for black communities in comparison to white elders of the same age.

Household composition

The lower rate of pensioner only households amongst black communities identified by the 1991 Census, inevitably disguises some degree of variance amongst the constituent part of the black communities. Some studies have explored this further. A study of black older people in London and Manchester by Barker (1984) showed that older people of Afro-Caribbean origin had a living situation similar to that of older white people living in the same inner city areas: 36 per cent lived on their own, 32 per cent lived with only one other person and two per cent lived with six others. Asian older people by contrast were much more likely to live with large households, usually kin: five per cent lived on their own, 13 per cent with one other and 71 per cent lived with six others.

Both the Donaldson and Odell (1984) study and the Farrah (1986) study confirm these findings. Donaldson and Odell found that Asian older people were more likely to live in a multi-generational households (82 per cent - 573 people out of 726 people sampled - lived in a household with two or more generations), than their white counterparts. Farrah, looking at the needs of Afro-Caribbean elders, found that 28 per cent (30 people out of 109 people sampled) lived on their own, 46 per cent (50 people) with one other person; 11 per cent (12 people) lived with two or more people and 13 per cent (14 people) with four or more people.

Although a higher rate of multi-generation households is found among Asian older people in general, such households may have resulted from economic necessity rather than desire. This may be due to limited access to housing, or employment, or the fact that a number of these Asian elders are dependent on their relatives because one of their conditions of entry into this country is that they do not have access to public funds. Furthermore, rather than being a source of support to older people, they may be a source of family stress (Turnbull, 1985) or fail to prevent loneliness. Such households may also fail to provide vital care to the elderly particularly if children are out working, or preoccupied with home-based employment (Williams, 1990).

Given the low levels of awareness of services, their use and the inability of service providers to accommodate the specific needs of Asian older people, some studies conclude that the evidence suggests 'containment rather than care' (Lewando-Hundt and Grant, 1987). Turnbull (1985) in a study of black older people living in the London Borough of Greenwich notes that the 'maintenance of a traditional extended family pattern for the majority may hide the most vulnerable minority'. She further notes that 'even within the extended family setting there was often conflict and loneliness' (Turnbull, 1985:20). She argues that the role of the elderly immigrant to Britain in the family and community is uncertain; changing patterns of family life, different hopes and ambitions among the younger ethnic minority population and the ethos of life in a highly industrialised western country have all undermined the traditional powerful role of black older people. Comments like 'All my children are very good to me - if I need anything they help me' were balanced with 'We like the children - to see them - but they don't like to see us'; 'They are too busy to be seen'. The sense of isolation and insecurity was exacerbated by language difficulties for many Asian older people, who had to rely on the family for translation.

The studies further show that for those who are not in multi-generational households, it cannot be assumed that they have an 'extended' family network nearby. Whereas about a quarter of Fenton's (1986) Asian older respondents lived in 'extended' households, three fifths lived in households described as 'nuclear'. A sizeable proportion of these latter respondents did not have the compensatory support of extended families in Bristol or even in the United Kingdom, either from choice, or because of immigration law, or financial barriers to the reunification of families.

Barker (1984:9) gives examples through case studies of black older people where there is very little contact outside the immediate family:

> Mrs P, a Ugandan Asian refugee, aged 78, widow, who lives on her own. She has no local friends nor any real contact with friends or kin in Gujarat or East Africa. All but one of her five children have emigrated to Canada. The remaining son, now in his fifties, lives in North London with his wife, mother and father in law and four children . . . Her only recent opportunity to meet other Asian people has been when she was ill and received visits from her son and local religious leaders . . .

Using snapshot surveys or data sources to examine dynamic relationships such as household compositions and the operations of extended family networks is inevitably problematic. However these studies do suggest that while multi-generational households may still be the norm for most black communities, we should not assume that they are either a source of support for black elders or able to provide for the care needs of these people. The evidence appears to suggest containment rather than care and certainly undermines the old adage that they look after their own.

Employment, pensions and poverty

Many of the studies on the health and social care needs of black older people provide evidence of higher levels of poverty amongst black older people. Few of the studies use a standard assessment of poverty and therefore it is difficult to compare the findings over time. But they do paint a consistent picture of financial hardship accompanied by stress.

Farrah (1986), for example, found that four in five people were living on incomes of less than £60 a week. Farrah further found that 77 per cent of the sample had difficulty managing on their current incomes, 24 per cent were struggling with food bills, 71 per cent paying gas bills and 66 per cent with electricity bills. Bhalla and Blakemore (1981:18) provide supporting evidence in that they found that old white people are more likely to have earned more throughout their working lives than blacks, to have benefited from an occupational pension, insurance scheme or interest on savings and to have, in retirement, a higher weekly income. Berry et al (1981) also found that of two thirds of those who were of pensionable age the State Retirement Pension was the main source of income and of the 97 people past retirement age, 81 were receiving a State Retirement Pension; 45 of these (56 per cent) were also receiving supplementary benefits.

A more recent study by Jadeja and Singh (1993) similarly found that most black older people in Britain today maintain themselves either on the level of income support rates or below the poverty level. They found that Asian older people had a weekly income of £59.10 a week whilst white older people had an income of £88.20 a week: a difference of £29.10 a week.

The financial position of black older people is often linked to the nature of their immigration into Britain as well as the opportunity to work so as to contribute to state or private pensions (Jadeja and Singh, 1993). The majority of black people who are presently experiencing poverty in retirement came to Britain through three main routes: firstly, refugees forced to leave former homes or colonies, like Ugandan Asians in the early 1970; secondly, elderly parents joining families who have settled in Britain; and thirdly, economic immigrants of the 1950s and 1960s. Those in the first two categories have had little opportunity to work and build state or private pensions. Those in the last category came to Britain when they were mainly in the middle of their working lives. They invariably came from countries with no state pension arrangements; they could only start contributing towards their pensions once they arrived in Britain. This left insufficient time to build any significant pensions (Barker, 1984; Farrah, 1986; Jadeja and Singh, 1993). This is reflected in the Jadeja and Singh (1993) survey, which showed that in the case of black older people 14 per cent had an occupational or state pension but the majority, 86 per cent, relied on income support. In comparison, within the white sample only 2 per cent did not have a state pension. Further, only 18 to 25 per cent of the white sample relied on or had their income topped up by income support.

Farrah's examination of the State Earnings Related Pension Scheme also showed that 'as most black elderly people came to Britain (between the ages of 29-49) they had not had enough years of National Insurance contributions to receive a full state pension' (Farrah, 1986: 20). Farrah shows that, of the 109 black older people interviewed, 60 per cent were in receipt of supplementary benefit, 54 per cent of State Earnings Related Pension and 24 per cent of both. Knowledge and take up of additional benefits and single payments was very low. For instance, 45 per cent had not heard of heating addition and 81 per cent were not claiming this, though a high proportion of the sample reported struggling with payment of gas bills and keeping the house warm. Farrah also found that a large proportion of the black older people participating in the study had suffered long periods of unemployment before reaching retirement, and only 7.3 per cent (eight people) were in employment at retirement. Ill health and racial discrimination were the most frequent reasons given for giving up work or for refusal of work: for example, 27 per cent reported ill health. In addition 19 per cent reported being refused employment because of racist employers, and of these three quarters were refused two or more times. The experience of racial harassment in employment is also noted by Turnbull (1985).

Clearly employment or lack of it is another contributing factor to the financial problems faced by black older people. The pattern of black employment in low paid jobs, often in the manufacturing sector, in unstable markets like textiles, heavy industries and semi-skilled machine tool manufacture is well documented. Donaldson and Odell (1984), for example, found that only 31 per cent of the Asian older people participating in their study had worked since they came to Britain. Of these 65 per cent had worked in unskilled manual occupations. Barker (1984) found that, although Afro-Caribbeans in his study had adequate income, no group of black older people was well off. Barker concludes that the reason for the difference is due to the earlier arrivals of Afro-Caribbeans in Britain and the fact that they tended to work for public employers, where contributions for those in employment were therefore paid on a regular basis. 'Asians, by contrast, were less likely to work for such responsible employers' (Barker, 1984: 24).

To summarise, the evidence demonstrates that black older people are likely to have a lower income than white older people. Indeed, Owen (1994d:9) in his analysis of the 1991 Census notes that the fact that 'more than half of all households headed by persons from each of the three Black ethnic groups do not possess a car compared to a third of white headed households' strongly indicates that black households have much lower income levels than white households. Further, their receipt of pensions is low, since these pensions are generally linked to type of occupation, stability of employment and final salary. For the majority, therefore, income in older age is made up by significant amounts of means-tested benefits.

Housing

Poor housing and inappropriate basic facilities is documented by many of the studies surveyed. Berry et al (1981) found that only 7.5 per cent of respondents lived in accommodation likely to be suitable for the elderly (bungalow and ground floor flat); the rest (one in five) lived in flats above ground floor level. Furthermore, 89 per cent of the sample lived within the inner city area and 87 per cent of these lived in the seven city wards which were defined as the 'worst' in Nottinghamshire in the 1975 County Deprived Area Study. Similarly, Bhalla and Blakemore (1981) found that a quarter of Asian older people lived in a house with no piped hot water as compared with 15 per cent of Europeans. Barker (1984) also found that overcrowding was a problem for many of the Asian older people participating in his study. Turnbull (1985) concludes that though it is difficult to make comparisons because of the small sample size the comments by participants reveal an element of dissatisfaction with their housing condition. She notes that comments with regard to housing ranged from:

> 'a wish for more space - a common plea, perhaps indicating the overcrowding known to exist in many Asian homes - through quite detailed lists of necessary home improvements 'rewiring, plastering, old windows and doors in the basement to be changed, ventilation to be properly made' to a now classic complaint about council flats 'It is the 7th floor, if the lift is not working it is very hard for me to climb the stairs'. (Turnbull, 1985:23)

Owen's analysis of the 1991 Census supports the findings above which suggest that Black older people are more likely to be found in older housing with fewer amenities (see our discussion in chapter 2, page 25).

Poor housing conditions have two consequences for black elders. Firstly, housing conditions do impact on the health of elderly people and the discussion in chapter 2 shows some evidence of the negative impact of poor housing. Second, home ownership is a valuable resource in older age as has been indicated through equity release schemes. However owning the worst types of accommodation severely limits what wealth black older people can draw upon.

Knowledge and use of services

Much of the available literature demonstrates lack of knowledge and under use of social care services by black older people irrespective of age and disability. A survey of black older people in Coventry by Lewando-Hundt and Grant (1987) looking at their present and future needs found that black older people knew very little about the social services available to them. Questions related to six areas of social services: mobile meals, home helps, sheltered housing, day centres, luncheon clubs and residential homes. The survey found that half of them did not know about any of the services, 45 per cent knew about some of them and only five per cent knew about all of them. Despite the health needs of the respondents a low proportion of black older people were in receipt of social services: for example, one per cent of the sample of Asians said that they used home helps and sheltered housing and four per cent said they used luncheon clubs. Afro-Caribbean older people also had low percentages in relation to use of social services. For example, three per cent used sheltered housing, eight per cent home helps, 22 per cent luncheon clubs and 32 per cent day centres.

Donaldson and Odell (1984), in a study examining the health and social services needs of Asian older people in Leicester, similarly found that few Asian older people were in receipt of certain social services which are normally provided for the elderly (for example meals on wheels, home help, social worker and day centre). Further, between 50 per cent and 70 per cent had not heard of these (between 641 and 715 people respectively).

Lewando-Hundt and Grant's (1987) finding that Afro-Caribbean older people were better informed about social services than Asian older people is reproduced in Table 9. The slightly higher use of services by the Afro-Caribbean older people, suggest the authors, may be a reflection of the differences in household composition and age structure.

Table 9 Black elders' knowledge of services - Lewando-Hundt and Grant

Services	Asians		Caribbeans	
	n	%	n	%
Mobile meals	163	14	62	87
Home helps	183	16	61	86
Sheltered housing	130	11	45	63
Day centres	530	46	67	94
Luncheon clubs	60	5	57	80
Residential homes	86	7	62	87

Source: Lewando-Hundt and Grant (1987:4).

However although Afro-Caribbeans appears to be better informed than Asians, their knowledge of social services is still lower than that for the white community (Bhalla and Blakemore, 1981; McCalman, 1990). Bhalla and Blakemore (1981) showed that white Europeans were consistently more aware of social services compared to both Asians and Afro-Caribbeans: see Table 10.

Table 10   Black elders' knowledge of services - Bhalla and Blakemore

Services	Asian % age	Afro-Caribbean % age	Europeans % age
Old people's home	33	89	96
Home helps	19	83	94
Meals-on-wheels	13	80	96
Day centres	13	60	67
Luncheon clubs	5	36	42
Night watch	4	23	36
Home visiting service for old people	11	58	62
None of these	3	64	2

Source: Bhalla and Blakemore (1981).

A similar picture emerges in terms of health services. Despite the greater use of GPs who might have been expected to be important sources of referral to other services, there is evidence to show a low level of contact with district nurses and health visitors among black older people (see above). When we go beyond primary care and consider out-patient clinics and residential facilities, the picture is no different. Blakemore (1982), for example, found that despite a high incidence of GP consultations, 99 per cent of Asian and 97 per cent of Afro-Caribbean elderly people had never seen a health visitor, while 99 per cent and 92 per cent respectively had never seen a district nurse.

Fenton (1986) also found that whilst higher percentages of Afro-Caribbean (75 per cent) and Asian (70 per cent) older people had visited their GPs recently, somewhat higher percentages of white older people had visited hospital in the last month and in the last year. Fenton notes, though this cannot be taken as conclusive evidence allowing for age and illness, white older people were making more use of services beyond primary care. Similar findings on low uptake of social and community health services were also reported by some of the other studies in this field (Bhalla and Blakemore, 1981; Donaldson, 1986; Boneham, 1989; and Evers et al, 1988).

Barriers

Two important barriers have been documented by a number of studies in relation to low level of knowledge and take up by black older people. These relate to access to information and the appropriateness of services provided. Atkin et al (1989) found that Asian older people said that they might be interested in using services if important provisos concerning cultural and religious needs were taken into account: the provision of vegetarian and halal meals on wheels and same sex bath nurses, for instance. They suggest services were often rejected because they were inappropriate, as in the case of two Asian women who terminated district nursing bath services because they found them inappropriate in that the style of provision did not meet with their requirements concerning rinsing. Similarly Lewando-Hundt and Grant (1987) found that interest in use of services in the future was qualified by a fairly widespread wish for meals which reflect the dietary preferences of black older people, home helps who are of the same ethnic origin, housing developments, day centres and luncheon clubs which are local and are attended by others of a similar background.

In a report of four projects concerned with the development and delivery of services to black and minority ethnic older people, Bowling (in Morton, 1992) notes that:

> The experience of Afro-Caribbean and Asian older people was that mainstream services were often neither accessible nor appropriate to their needs. Project workers found that there was little or no commitment to plan for further needs of these groups as they aged, despite the fact that the population was growing apace rather than dying off. For many service providers coming into contact with these projects, the idea that black older people might be a significant social group or that they might face specific problems had come as something of a revelation. (Bowling, in Morton, 1992:6)

The reason given as to why social services departments were reluctant to develop services for them related to things like low numbers; for example, a social services official from Northampton said 'At the moment numbers do not justify the extra provision', despite trends which show that the proportion of black older people is increasing not only nationally but locally in Northampton. Bowling concludes that until adequate, appropriate and accessible services are provided and effort is made to publicise these, take up will always be low. If this is not acted upon 'we will be deliberately allowing many black older people to grow old in fear and isolation and to die of untreated illness, malnutrition and lack of care' (Bowling in Morton, 1992:8).

A study by Askham (1995) asked black older people how they wanted to be treated when receiving health and social care services. The study found that a higher proportion of Asian older people said they wanted to be treated in a 'special' way (40 per cent - 36 people out of a sample of 89 people). When the evidence was analysed in more detail, the study revealed that being treated in a 'special' way related to having a need for specific services or types of care such as language and food. For example, a 52 year old Asian woman said 'Yes, we want more nurses who speak our language and more understanding about our culture. We are human too. Our needs are the same as anybody's. When you go into a place where you can't speak or understand they must be patient and teach us what to do' (Askham et al, 1995:84).

The Afro-Caribbean respondents on the other hand did not express a desire to be treated in a 'special' way but to be treated fairly, kindly and effectively. Detailed analysis of comments made reveals that the stress on equality was an important factor. For example, a 70 year old Afro-Caribbean woman said 'I don't think people should be treated differently on grounds of ethnic origin. All people should be treated equal according to their individual needs' (Askham et al, 1995:80). Askham et al note that 'in referring to equality they called upon common characteristics such as common humanity, being a member of the British family or a British citizen, one of God's children, or a tax-payer' (Askham et al, 1995:79).

The study further noted that the lack of interpreting facilities at hospitals (both in-patient and out-patient) contributed difficulties to access and uptake for Asian older people. For example, when asked if interpreting was offered over half said no. Family and friends were often the source of interpreting: in Askham et al's study 57 per cent (51 people) used the family while over a quarter(27 per cent - 24 people) used friends. As importantly, language was often highlighted as being a factor in relation to accessibility of services, echoing other studies (Barker, 1984; Prime, 1987; Donaldson and Odell, 1984; Atkin et al, 1989; Bowling, 1990.)

Specific or separate services

A number of studies recently have examined the extent of specific or separate services for black people. The evidence suggest that there is very little in the way of specific or even separate provision that is appropriate to the needs of black older people. The lack of services for black older people exists despite the very significant numbers of black people in the population. For example, in a study of home help and home care services in four local authorities in London, Gorbach (1989) found that only one authority had a rate of cover for black clients even approaching that for white clients despite the fact that 'all four authorities had significant black elderly populations even by the 1981 Census classification' (Gorbach, 1989:2).

Askham et al (1995) in a survey of social services departments (SSDs) and district health authorities (DHAs) with a significant proportion of black older people found that very few specific and even fewer separate services existed. They note that 'service provision for elderly people from black and minority ethnic groups appeared to vary considerably, both between the various services and between different departments' (Askham et al, 1995:35). So much so that it was not possible to discern how such services came into being, nor their operation or their likely future.

The study found that residential care was the least likely to cater in a specific or separate way for such groups: two thirds of the departments responding to the survey offered only mainstream services in this area. Home help/care services came next, with one third of the departments offering only mainstream services, and only one having access to a separate service for people from black communities. However, for day centres, lunch clubs and meals on wheels, most departments said they were able to offer some specific or separate provision; half funded or ran separate day centres, and two-thirds ran or funded separate or specific meals on wheels services or lunch clubs. Askham et al (1995:35) note that 'this does not, however, mean either that such provision was on a wide scale within the area covered by the department or that it was necessarily considered a wholly desirable form of service delivery. It was clear that even departments which had made efforts to cater for the specific needs of service users from at least some black and minority ethnic groups were only providing such services on a very small scale'. Indeed, they continue that much of the scant provision available is non-local authority service run either with full or partial statutory sector funding.

The study further found that the views of the majority of social services and health authority staff, at all levels, was that the absence of specific services was unsatisfactory. Most did not want to see separate provision (except for day care) but did want specific needs to be catered for.

Pharoah (in Morton, 1992) similarly found that most primary care providers perceived the level of care provided directly or indirectly to black older people as unsatisfactory. Most of those participating in the study felt that they could not give black older people's needs priority. To this extent certain inadequacies were even tolerated. This was especially evident in relation to the over 75s health checks, where GP respondents often noted high levels of difficulty in proper assessment while also reporting that they had installed few specific measures to address those needs. Walker and Ahmad (1994), in a report of a survey of care providers' perspectives on the implications of community care policy for black older people in Bradford, make a pertinent point: they note that there was a consensus amongst partici-pants that the statutory services are ill equipped to meet the needs of black older people. Participants perceived this to be because, in part, of stereotypical thinking about black older people and in part, of fear of uncovering needs which would call resource allocations into question.

Conclusion

The studies reviewed here, though small scale and local, demonstrate that considerable health and social care needs exist amongst black older people. While the evidence on intensity is sketchy, it is clear that the inability to perform some basic tasks affects a comparatively younger group of black older people than white older people. Some may have argued that the small numbers of black elderly people indicated a lower priority for developing appropriate services. However the growth of the black pensioner population by 168% suggests at the very least the need for greater urgency.

Though the proportion of 'pensioner only' households is low amongst black older people, the family and household structures of black older people are not homogenous. Equally, the fact that a higher proportion of black older people live in multi-generational households does not mean that they have no needs since their needs are being met by the extended family network, as a number of studies suggest: the evidence points as much to containment as care. The literature also suggests that black older people are more likely to have lower incomes than white older people and live in poorer housing that lacks basic amenities.

Common to all of the research reviewed here has been the low level of knowledge about services and under use by black older people. Issues relating to accessibility, appropriateness and communication have been identified as the main barriers to under use of existing services by black older people.

5

Mental health

Summary

This chapter explores black communities' experience of the mental health system in England. It does not explore definitions of mental illness or mental well-being in any depth, except to note that there is an increasing recognition that attention must be paid to the possible cultural specificity of western notions of mental illness and that failure to do so may have a negative impact on responding to the needs of black communities.

The chapter then considers compulsory detention of people of Caribbean and Asian origin. We consider the Caribbean community first. The studies vary in their findings as to whether it is first or second generation people of Caribbean origin who are over-represented, or whether it is the young or older people from this community who are over-represented, or whether it is men or women. However, they are consistent in showing some form of over- representation of the Caribbean community under a compulsory order, most suggesting that this is particularly so for young men. There is further evidence of over-representation in secure units and some suggestion that those held in these units are less likely to have committed serious offences and more likely to have been referred because they have absconded rather than because they are deemed aggressive.

The evidence with regard to the Asian community is contradictory, in that some studies suggest over-representation in admissions while others suggest rates similar to the English, while others suggest under-representation. The evidence on admission is accompanied by contradictory evidence about mental illness and the rates of diagnosed schizophrenia, leading one commentator to conclude that the experience of Asians is the opposite of Afro-Caribbeans. At present we can only conclude that there are Asian people in the mental health system and that some of them are being compulsorily detained. Whether their patterns of admission indicate the operation of discrimination is unclear.

In examining access to services and treatment there is some evidence that black people do not have access to counselling services and psychotherapy. One study suggests that they are more likely to be put on drug regimes and that compulsory entry to hospital is the most likely outcome for people of Afro-Caribbean origin after Approval Social Worker assessment.

Research on mental health and black communities has seen the conjuncture of several disciplines: psychiatry, psychology, sociology, anthropology, genetics, human biology. A constant theme, however, has been the attempt to explain differences between the experience of black and white people of mental health services provided by the state in pathological terms. This chapter only briefly covers the large number of studies which have tried to explain the apparently differing patterns of mental illness between black and white communities. Detailed discussions have been provided by Mercer (1986), Francis (1991) and most recently, amongst others. Of more concern to us in this chapter is exploring the presence (or the lack of presence) of black people in the mental health system, their route of entry and their experience once in the system.

Before discussing these issues three points need to be noted. First, the mental health system in England covers a wide spectrum of services from those provided privately drawing on a wide range of counselling techniques, to secure mental health institutions operated by central government. However, the debate about services to black communities has been dominated by their experience of the services that fall in the latter part of the spectrum. Second, the debate has most often identified over-representation of the Caribbean community in compulsory detention and has therefore concentrated on attempting to provide an explanation for this situation. This has sometimes meant that results for Asian people are not always presented. However, this situation may be changing (Ineichen, 1990:1669).

Third, almost all the studies are cross-sectional and rarely deal with experience over time. This has led to a static view of black communities' experience of mental health services. For example, even though some of Cope's (1989) work covers admissions over an eight year period there is no presentation of data that change over time. As a result we are unable to assess changes such as the impact of growing numbers of black professionals in the mental health system or the growth in black self-help groups. Equally we are unable to explore whether the differences in experience of the Caribbean community in comparison to the Asian community may be partly explained by their length of exposure to the British mental health system. The consequence of these three points is that the literature has several important gaps.

Concepts of mental illness

An essential element in discussing black people and mental health must be some conception of what constitutes mental well-being as well as what constitutes mental illness. For many of the studies that have explored mental illness in black communities there has been no attempt to explore what this actually means to black communities themselves (Webb-Johnson, 1991:19). Beliappa, drawing on the commentaries of Fernando and others, notes in her study on mental health in the Asian community:

> The report attempts to reach conceptualisations of mental health as it is defined by the community. Accordingly, classifications such as 'mental-illness' and 'depression' derived from the western medical model are treated with caution. Emotional disturbances are traditionally described as 'sorrow', 'anxiety' or as a 'burden' and therefore are not seen as pathological within Asian cultures. The absence of an equivalent South Asian term for depression raises interesting questions on certain assumptions about normality.
>
> Differences in the way emotions are expressed and dealt with vary across cultures and are a function of the cultural shaping of normative and deviant behaviour. The 'depressive syndrome' for example is a category of symptoms developed by psychiatrists to yield a homogeneous group of patients . . . To apply this as a universal tool would possibly lead to the danger of over-generalisation of 'symptoms' that may not be relevant for cultural groups with different notions of pathological behaviour. On the other hand, symptoms that do not fit easily into these parameters could easily be missed . . . (Beliappa, 1991:2)

Some have begun to consider the possible implications of this lack of understanding. Reed (1994) in the Department of Health/Home Office review of services to mentally disordered offenders concluded:

> The lack of basic knowledge about the needs of minority ethnic communities and poor understanding of institutional racism noted by the MHAC [Mental Health Act Commission] raised questions about how the differing needs of minority communities are met in hospital. It does not appear that consideration has often been given to the relationship between the alleged lack of co-operation by the patient and lack of knowledge and understanding by the staff. Little is done to

ensure that the patients' concepts of mental health are listened to and respected. (Reed, 1994:14)

For many of the studies however there has been an acceptance of western definitions of mental illness and the use of particular symptoms to indicate diseases such as schizophrenia. This has often continued in the face of critiques forwarded in the west about the role of psychiatry in controlling the 'troublesome' and in defining who is dangerous (Francis, 1991:85-87), with critics such as Thomas Szasz suggesting schizophrenia was little more than an 'exercise in labelling' (quoted by Ineichen, 1989:335). Inevitably, it appears that studies spend more time considering why their evidence indicates higher rates of mental illness in black (most often Caribbean) communities than whether it is their diagnosis which is wrong. As a result we have had a multitude of explanations forwarded in support of the greater propensity to diagnose psychosis from perinatal illnesses, to genetic defects, to socio-economic stress, to the impact of racism, to a combination of all of these.

Cope (1989:351) in discussing her findings notes these criticisms but suggests that there have been no alternative diagnostic criteria suggested. Nevertheless, the failure of most studies to examine their notions of mental illness does suggest that we should see these studies as illustrating whether or not black people are in contact with the system rather than use them as an indication of the prevalence of mental illness in black communities (Grimley and Bhatt, 1989:194).

Compulsory detention

Research evidence on experience of black communities of the controlling end of the mental health system is the most plentiful. However, it is worth presenting separately the evidence for people of Caribbean origin and those of Asian origin.

Caribbean people

While the evidence from different studies is not always comparable it has led Francis to conclude that there is now consensus on this evidence (if not why this situation has come about) (Francis, 1991:81). Francis summarises the evidence thus:

British-born 'Afro-Caribbeans' are more likely than 'white' Britons to be:

- diagnosed as suffering from schizophrenia and less likely to be diagnosed as suffering from depression (Harrison et al, 1988);

- referred to hospital under compulsory procedures of the Mental Health Act 1983 (Cope, 1989);

- referred to psychiatric hospital with the involvement of police under Section 136 of the Mental Health Act (Rogers and Faulkner, 1987);
- referred to hospital by a court order under Section 37 of the Mental Health Act or be classified as a restricted patient under Section 41 (Browne 1990);
- referred from prison to a special hospital or regional secure unit under Section 47 for remandees and Section 48 for convicted offenders (Cope and Ndegwa, 1991);
- treated with large psychotic medication (Littlewood and Cross, 1980).

(Francis, 1991:82-83)

This summary of studies published in the 1980s to some extent counters Cochrane's findings in the 1970s. Cochrane's analysis of the 1971 hospital admissions had suggested that while West Indians immigrants were much more likely than their white (and other immigrant) counterparts to be diagnosed schizophrenic (290 per 100,000 as opposed to 98 per 100,000) they were in fact not over-represented in hospitals when standardised for age and sex (Cochrane, 1977).

The picture is, however, slightly more complex than that suggested by Francis' summary. Francis has attempted to draw together only that evidence which is comparable across all the studies. Many of the studies do additionally provide some information on gender differences and age, as well as possible differences between first and second generation migrants.

Cope (with McGovern [1989]) carried out four studies of compulsory detention under the Mental Health Acts (their data collection encompassed the transition from the 1958 Mental Health Act to the 1983 Mental Health Act) in Birmingham and she was able to explore both Part II admissions (civil commitments) and Part III (forensic sections). Her Tables 1 and 2 are reproduced here as Table 11 and Table 12 below. She notes that with regard to Part II admissions the greatest disparity between Afro-Caribbeans and whites is in the 16 to 29 age range, with migrant Afro-Caribbeans having an admission rate 17 times that of their white counterparts (p346). A similar but more stark picture emerges with Part III detention rates, with young migrant Afro-Caribbeans having a rate that is twenty-five times that of their white counterparts. She suggests that further statistical analysis points to this over-representation in compulsory detention under Part II and Part III being explained by Afro-Caribbean over-representation in total admissions (p347).

Table 11 Part II four-year detention rates per 10,000 population at risk

	Age 16-29	Age 30-44	Age 45-65
White	8.8	12.8	12.4
Afro-Caribbean migrant	148.8	87.4	19.6
British Afro-Caribbean	77.9	34.6	18.6

Source: Cope (1989:346) Table 1.

Table 12 Part III eight-year detention rates per 10,000 population at risk

	Age 16-29	Age 30-44	Age 45-65
White	3.7	5.6	1.6
Afro-Caribbean migrant	90.9	38.3	19.6
British Afro-Caribbean	16.4	-	-

Source: Cope (1989:346) Table 2.

Continuing her analysis of compulsory detention, Cope then presents a series of other studies involving an examination of first admissions only, first admissions with a psychotic diagnosis and admissions to a secure unit. Cope shows that the diagnosis of psychosis is higher for both migrant and British-born young Afro-Caribbean males in comparison to whites (82 per cent, 92 per cent and 49 per cent respectively) with a similar picture emerging for young women (76 per cent for Afro-Caribbean migrants, 88 per cent for British-born Afro-Caribbeans and 44 per cent for whites) (Cope, 1989:348-349).

Her analysis of those who were in two secure units at the time of her study suggested that the source of referral was significantly different, with 91 per cent of Afro-Caribbeans coming from prisons as opposed to 54 per cent of whites. When looking just at offender patients in these secure units a 'significantly' smaller proportion of Afro-Caribbeans than whites were charged with serious offences (p350). She further notes that more Afro-Caribbeans were referred to the secure units rather than their local hospital because they absconded and not because they were aggressive.

Clearly, care must be taken with studies such as Cope's, particularly in terms of rates of psychotic diagnosis which we have already suggested has come under scrutiny for its possible cultural specificity. In addition Sashidharan (1988) has questioned the dependency of these rates on the accuracy of the 1981 Census in counting the number of Afro-Caribbeans in Britain. Under-counting by the 1981 Census would lead to higher rates. To which we must add some concern about how people involved in these studies have had their ethnicity classified: it appears to have been done in most cases by the researchers examining case records.

Nevertheless, this study does tell us about what happens to people of Caribbean origin. Once they are actually involved with the system they are much more likely to be held compulsorily, particularly young men and probably young women too. Being born in Britain does not lead to less representation under a compulsory order, as may have been expected if this migrant community was to display the patterns of other migrant communities (Mercer, 1986:113). Those held under the most controlling regimes (secure units) are less likely to have committed serious offences and less likely to have been described as aggressive. In addition to the studies quoted by Francis above (see page 74) this picture is confirmed by a number of studies: for example Bolton in his study of admissions in a fifteen month period in one psychiatric hospital found that West Indian and African compulsorily detained patients were four times more likely than white patients to be transferred to a 'high security unit' (Bolton, 1984 as quoted by Cope, 1989:344).

Asians

The picture for the Asian community is less confused. Some studies have either not focused on this community or do so only in passing (for example Cope, 1989). Of greater significance is that the evidence has often been contradictory. Cochrane (1977) suggested that the admission rate for Indian and Pakistani immigrants was lower than that for the English and Caribbean migrants. Grimley and Bhatt quote work carried out by Dean et al (1981) which showed higher admissions rates for Indian men and women, but lower rates for Pakistani men and women than the English (Grimley and Bhatt, 1989:194). However, Hitch (1981) suggested significantly higher admission rates for Pakistani women and lower rates for Indian women then their British counterparts (Hitch, 1981:).

This contradictory evidence is also reflected in debates about diagnosis. Ineichen suggests that there is evidence that less mental illness is 'found' amongst most groups of British Asians than might be expected (Ineichen, 1990:1669). However Grimley and Bhatt note Cochrane's findings that Indians and Pakistanis were one-and-a-half times more likely to be diagnosed as schizophrenic than their white counterparts. They quote other studies (Dean et al, 1981; Carpenter and Brockington, 1980) which also show higher rates of diagnosed schizophrenia amongst both Asian men and women (Grimley and Bhatt, 1989:195). However, all show rates of diagnosis of schizophrenia for Asians that are lower than their Caribbean counterparts. Francis, drawing on the work on Beliappa, goes further. He suggests that the experience of Asians is virtually the opposite to that of Afro-Caribbeans, with 'Asians under-represented in most services' (Francis, 1991:82). Cope, however, in her one reference to

Asians notes that results for them were similar to those for whites (Cope, 1989:345).

Ineichen, in a review of literature that considers the whole of the mental health field, notes:

> Although Asians may thus show both genuinely low rates of mental illness and a tendency to under-report mental illness, their prevalence of mental illness will probably gradually reach national levels, both overall and for particular diagnoses. (Ineichen, 1990:1670)

Asians, Caribbeans and ASW assessment

Bowl and Barnes' (1990) study provides further comparisons between Asian and Afro-Caribbean people. However, this work differs from many of the studies quoted previously as it is the result of the monitoring of all referrals for Approved Social Worker assessment in 10 social services departments, rather than an examination of case records of people in hospital already. After qualifying their results, Bowl and Barnes note that referral for ASW assessment was 116.7 per 100,000 for the whole population but that for Afro-Caribbeans was 204 per 100,000 and 54.3 per 100,000 for Asians.

When they consider outcomes (whether as a result of ASW assessment people were compulsorily detained, persuaded to enter informally, or there was an alternative outcome) they note that 'Afro-Caribbeans were most likely to be compulsorily detained, particularly after assessment for emergency admission.' Asian people and white people, however, often had similar outcomes: for example 59% of white people and 58.3% of Asian people were compulsorily detained. Nevertheless when age was taken into account (they present their results in terms of those under 35 or those over 35) they show compulsory admission rates for Asian young men similar to those of Afro-Caribbean young men (61.7 per cent and 63.2 per cent respectively). They further note that Asian women's compulsory admission is lower than for all other men and women, but informal admission of young Asian women is higher than for all other young men and women (Bowl and Barnes, 1990:14).

Doubts expressed about the methodology of studies with regard to the Caribbean community are equally relevant to those studies that have looked at the Asian community. However, it is possible to suggest that the experience of Asians of the 'harder end' of the British mental health system is different from that of the Caribbean community: they do not appear to be over-represented to the same extent. Furthermore they do not appear to be diagnosed as schizophrenic with the same regularity as their fellow immigrants. Importantly, there is also some evidence of a higher rate of informal admission for young Asian women.

How much these differences are due to differences in incidence of mental illness, or how much this is explained by other variables such as differences in contact with the state services, remains unclear. Bowl and Barnes (1990) do recount the view of practitioners that although the Asian community suffers similar racism to Afro-Caribbeans their socio-economic status and their family and religious support systems may cushion them and allow them to contain and absorb the effects of racism, resulting in lower referrals rates for compulsory detention assessments (Bowl and Barnes, 1990:13). They proceed to support this view by reference to high levels of owner-occupation and incidence of living alone amongst Asians as opposed to Afro-Caribbeans.

We have already noted, however, that high levels of owner-occupation amongst Asians disguise the fact that they actually live in the poorest quality owner-occupied housing available (see chapter 2). Furthermore, the propensity for living alone is an inadequate indicator of the support networks that can be drawn upon. This would be better assessed by looking at who people meet and how often, as well as what each relationship provides in terms of support. It is likely that the practitioners' views that Bowl and Barnes quote, tells us more about the stereotypical views held by the practitioners than offer any assessment of the networks of support that various black communities can draw upon.

To summarise, black communities do appear to be over-represented in the compulsory or secure end of the British mental health system. There is some variation in the rates of over-representation of the different constituent parts of black communities, with some studies noting age, gender, as well as whether the person was born in Britain as important variables. Variation also appears to occur between people of Caribbean origin and those of Asian origin. The picture with regard to Asian people is particularly contradictory with studies showing both over-representation as well as under-representation, particularly in compulsory detention, but possibly in the diagnosis of schizophrenia too.

Access and treatment

The differing experience of compulsory detention between black and white people is also reflected in access to various forms of treatment. Beliappa in her descriptive study of 92 Asian people in Haringey suggests that there is a lack of awareness of where to go when confronted with 'emotional distress': she noted that only 6 per cent were aware that support from social workers was a possibility

(Beliappa, 1991:73). While there was some evidence of GPs being used, it was often to deal with the physical consequences of emotional distress rather than the emotional distress (see Webb-Johnson's [1991:21] summary of Beliappa). Webb-Johnson (1991) suggests that Fenton and Sadiq show a similar picture in terms of willingness to use western medicine to treat the physical ailments, but uncertainty about its ability to deal with the 'classic symptoms' of depression. Beliappa suggests that alternatives appear to be used at times, including religious prayer and spiritual healers (Webb-Johnson, 1991:21).

Baylies et al (1993) paint a similar - but more detailed - picture to that of Beliappa, but in this instance with a group of people who are already in contact with the mental health system. They report on a study of 101 black patients discharged from hospital between September 1st 1990 and August 31st 1991, 63 of their carers, plus several voluntary organisations in Leeds and Bradford. They note low take up of and knowledge of community services among patients, although three quarters were in contact with GPs. Importantly they suggest that 80% had not seen a social worker or a CPN prior to their latest admission, even though the majority had already been in hospital at least once (Baylies et al, 1993:7). Much of the experience detailed by Baylies et al is reflected in the inquiry report on the care and treatment of Christopher Clunis, whose contact with community services was at best haphazard (Ritchie, 1994; also see Harris, 1994).

In addition their carers were also unsure about the services available (p8) and they appeared to be poorly supported (p10). Baylies et al proceed to discuss a number of factors that may impact on the use of hospital and community services including cultural and language barriers, services that meet the concerns of the users, difficulties with the location of some services, as well as poor integration of the specialist transcultural unit with other services for patients who had been discharged (p9). As with Beliappa, Baylies et al note the value of religious groups for some users (p8) and the impact of black-led voluntary support groups (p7).

In a different context Bowl and Barnes acknowledge the possible impact of black Approved Social Workers, but note that this is unlikely to have a major impact if alternative resources that are acceptable to black people are not available (Bowl and Barnes, 1990:16). A constant theme, however, in the findings of these various studies is the availability of services that are taken up by white people but not by black people.

Physical and non-physical treatment

Baylies et al also draw attention to their respondents' experience of counselling, in particular psychotherapy. After highlighting concern about the narrow range of services available they note:

> Most significantly, the experience of this sample is of limited availability of counselling and therapy services, both before and after discharge. A similar point was strongly argued by representatives of community groups. The deficiency is in large part attributable to the lack of resources, particularly qualified and appropriate staff, although there are also signs that black ethnic minority clients are not encouraged (or offered the opportunity in some instances) to explore this particular care route. (Baylies et al, 1993:10)

Bowl and Barnes record that three of the ten authorities involved in their in-depth work noted a concern that mental health services are not accessible enough to black people (Bowl and Barnes, 1990:13). Similarly, Mercer in his review of transcultural psychiatry draws attention to psychotherapy, suggesting either low take up of these services or low rates of referral to them (Mercer, 1986:124).

There is some evidence that treatment instead has focused on drug (or physical) regimes. Littlewood and Cross's study (quoted by Grimley and Bhatt, 1989:198) of outpatients in an East London general hospital showed black patients (West Indian, African and Asian) were more likely to be:

> receiving major tranquillisers than whites;
>
> receiving intra-muscular medication than whites;
>
> receive electroconvulsive-therapy without a diagnosis of depression.

They also found some evidence for higher than average doses for black people as opposed to white people, but suggested that this was the result of a small group of black patients receiving very high doses.

Little further evidence has been ascertained for this experience.[7] However, some evidence may be gleaned from the official enquiry that followed Orville Blackwood's death in Broadmoor Hospital on August 28th, 1991. The pathologist noted that the cause of death was 'cardiac failure associated with the administration of phenothiazine drugs' (quoted by Sheppard, 1995:11). Blackwood had voluntarily gone into a seclusion room on the day of his death and after a review that afternoon was restrained and injected with 150mg sparine and 150 mg modecate and died almost immediately (quoted by Sheppard, 1995:10). How common this experience is, is difficult to say.

Nevertheless it has led Francis to argue for a link between black people's experience of physical and non-physical treatment regimes. He suggests:

> The concentration of black patients in secure settings, which primarily use pharmacological and physical restraint as the main therapeutic tool, has led to the under-use of counselling, psychotherapy and group work. This reflects a vestigial form of the classical racist-scientific view that black people are incapable of experiencing depression and that their under-developed linguistic and intellectual faculties renders them unsuitable for psychotherapeutic treatment. In the absence of the appropriate use of these resources, black patients are put at a disadvantage; it is thus more difficult to obtain advance warning of crises. The eventual crises, often involving black individuals and families, may leave no alternative but for legal sanction (or some form of custodial option) to be exercised. (Francis, 1991:88)

Baylies et al (1993) do record that when black people viewed services as responding to their needs they were willing to use them.

Entering hospitals
An essential element in the debate on both the over-representation in compulsory detention as well as accessing supportive services has been how black people come into contact with the British mental health system. Some material already reviewed has suggested that GPs are an important entry point (Baylies et al, 1993; Beliappa, 1991). In the case of the Asian community they may be the point at which Asians are diverted away from other aspects of the British mental health system such as social workers, counselling and mental health institutions (Ineichen, 1990; Webb-Johnson, 1991; Bowl and Barnes, 1990). However, other points of entry have been highlighted too: the police; the wider criminal justice system; and Approved Social Worker assessment.

Mercer has noted the shift in admissions to hospital since the 1950s, which has seen a dramatic decline in compulsory admission (which was the norm in the 1930s) to a situation where voluntary admission is now the 'norm' (Mercer, 1986:14) even though there are a number of compulsory powers still available to relatives, GPs, social workers and the police. However he highlights Littlewood and Lipsedge's (1982) findings with regard to the use of Section 136 (which empowers the police to hold in a place of safety any person who is seen in a public place and regarded to be a danger), noting that they showed black people were twice as likely as white people to be 'caught' by this aspect of the law. Grimley and Bhatt (1989:197) have summarised some of the studies in the 1980s that suggested a similar pattern, with black people (of Afro-Caribbean and Asian origin) being over-represented in compulsory admission under Section 136 (Ineichen et al, 1984; Hitch and Clegg, 1980; Rwegellera, 1980; Littlewood and Lipsedge, 1977); and Francis has summarised those for the latter part of the 1980s (Rogers and Faulkner, 1987) as well as others that detailed movements from within the criminal justice system to mental health institutions (Browne 1990; Cope and Ndegwa, 1991).

In exploring this question Bowl and Barnes (1990) have adopted a different strategy: they have attempted to look at source of referral and likely ASW outcome. Their analysis of source of referral is produced as their Table 1 and is reproduced here as Table 13. They firstly suggest that of their study areas only in London are black people over-represented in referrals under Section 136 and then 'only marginally' (p13). Furthermore, besides 'psychiatric services' the most likely sources of referrals were GPs for Asians and 'informal' (family, friends etc) for Afro-Caribbeans. In considering referral source with ASW outcome, they note:

> The group most likely to be detained - Afro-Caribbeans - are least often referred by sources identified . . . as most likely to pass on cases resulting in compulsory admission (the psychiatric services). They are most often referred by the sources least likely to lead to compulsory detention. The assessment by an ASW appears therefore to amplify the discriminatory effects of referral patterns, reinforcing the tendency for Afro-Caribbeans to be subject to compulsory detention. (Bowl and Barnes, 1990:14)

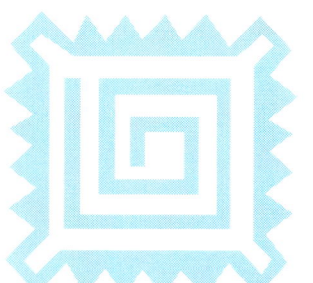

Table 13 Source of referral by ethnic group

	White	**Afro-Caribbean**	**Asian**
Informal	11.5	14.1	10.8
Police/Courts	8.5	10.0	7.6
GP	15.7	9.7	21.7
Psychiatric services	64.8	43.8	52.2
SSD	10.5	13.2	3.2

Source: Bowl and Barnes (1990:14) Table 1.

It appears, then, regardless of whether the past evidence of the use of Section 136 is contradicted by Bowl and Barnes, the outcome of compulsory detention is still prevalent for people of Afro-Caribbean origin, even when they are referred by family and friends. This may reflect the possibility that families and friends of Afro-Caribbean people are waiting until a crisis occurs which they cannot cope with, and therefore leaves no alternative but a compulsory admission after ASW assessment (Francis, 1991:88 quoted here on page 82). However, Bowl and Barnes do argue that there is no reason to suggest that one

group is more ill or in greater crisis than another at the time of referral, because the referrer already feels that compulsory admission is a
strong possibility (Bowl and Barnes, 1990:14). It is for this reason,
they argue, that the differing outcomes for Afro-Caribbeans who have
been informally referred is a product of the amplification of
discrimination.

Conclusion

Whether or not black people are in the mental health system as a
result of greater likelihood of illness or because of discrimination, it
is clear that they are certainly over-represented in the compulsory or
secure end, under a legal order. This is particularly so for those of
Afro-Caribbean origin. The evidence varies as to whether this is only
so for first generation (migrant) Afro-Caribbeans or second
generation (British born) Afro-Caribbeans. Also, there is some variance in terms of age and gender. The evidence for Asians is more
confused, with some studies suggesting similar patterns to white
people, while others demonstrate over-representation for Indians or
Pakistanis or young Asian men. However, Asians are less likely to be
diagnosed as schizophrenic then Caribbean people.

All black people appear to have some difficulty in accessing
counselling, including psychotherapy. This is probably due to a combination of factors: they are sent into that part of the system that is
more likely to use physical treatment; the counselling service is either
inadequate or inappropriate to their needs; or they are unaware of
the availability of these services. However, when these services are
available and appropriate there is evidence of use and a feeling
amongst black people that they are benefiting.

6

Disability

Summary

This chapter reviews the attempts to develop a theoretical frame-work to understand the experience of black disabled people. After noting the shift from seeing black disabled peoples' lives in terms of double discrimination (or jeopardy) to one which is of multiple and simultaneous oppression, we note that much of the research evidence has still not caught up with these debates. Much of it continues to think of disability in terms of physical or mental impairment rather than focusing on how society disables by not providing buses or buildings that are accessible. Inevitably, because of the dominance to date of this type of research, we have to draw our evidence for the incidence, prevalence and characteristics of social care needs from this material.

The studies focusing specifically on black disabled people suggest a higher incidence of impairment or disability than is true for their white counterparts. However this is not confirmed by evidence from the 1991 Census question on limiting long term illness. The chapter focuses on sensory and learning disability, identifying evidence of higher rates of impairment. This discussion also highlights the tendency to ignore causes of these disabilities forwarded when discussing the white majority community (poverty, housing, education) and to focus on pathological explanations such as first cousin marriages.

In exploring the experience of disability and attitudes towards disability in black communities, the chapter notes evidence of the intermingling of negative views of black people and disabled people, combined with negative attitudes within black communities. The chapter draws on evidence which demonstrates the negative consequences for black disabled people and their carers of these views, leading to a 'low' take up of services as well as ignorance of the existence of services or rejection of those that were taken up.

While there are a large number of commentaries and attempts to deal with the theoretical understanding in relation to disability (Begum, 1994) there has been little investigation into the extent and nature of disability among black people (see McAvoy and Donaldson, 1990; McDonald, 1991). Research and planning have often been preoccupied with specific problems such as rickets, osteomalacia, thalassaemia, sickle cell anaemia and tuberculosis (see Donovan, 1984; Brozovic et al, 1989; Balarajan and Bulusu, 1990). Atkin and Rollings (1993) argue that, although these diseases require specialised services, they affect relatively few people and deflect attention away from more widespread need.

However, over the last decade the number of studies assessing the incidence of disability in black people has slowly grown. Much of this, though, concentrates on disability in old age and physical disability (see Donaldson and Odell, 1984; Farrah, 1986; GLAD, 1987). In comparison to physical disability, there is little information on black people with learning difficulties or on people with hearing and visual impairments. Methodological issues further complicate the research. Data on the extent of problems associated with mental health, for example, are often problematic because of cultural bias in diagnosis and the effects of racism (see the discussion in chapter 5). Even less information is available on the relationship between black people's experience of health, illness, disability and the nature of community care services.

A related problem with reviewing this literature is that there are various definitions of disability used by the studies. This is not just a facet of research on black communities as there has been considerable debate about defining disability (Morris, 1995) with a call by the 'disability movement' to move away from a medical definition that focuses on the individual to one that focuses on how society disables by making buildings or transport or education inaccessible. One of the most significant demonstrations of these challenges has been Barnes' (1991) questioning of the findings of the 1987 OPCS survey of disability, focusing in particular on who was defined as disabled. The controversy sparked by the recent changes in the invalidity and sickness benefit regulations suggests that definitions remain contentious. For our review, we have tried not to impose a definition of disability on to the literature and have instead chosen to work with those definitions that the studies referred to here have used. This has meant various indicators of disability are used, particularly illness. However, we do explore how some writers have tried to conceptualise the experience of disability in black communities, and highlight the definitions of disability used by some of the studies quoted.

Double disadvantage and triple jeopardy

As is the case for black older people the concepts of 'double disadvantage' and 'triple jeopardy' have been forwarded to help understand black disabled people's lives. However, Begum (1994) argues that the notion of 'double disadvantage' or 'triple jeopardy' does nothing to facilitate understanding of multiple and simultaneous oppression experienced by black disabled people. She argues that multiple and simultaneous oppression are not lived out separately or in a hierarchical structure and thus they cannot be compartmentalised into neat discrete categories. She continues 'More importantly, such notions as "double disadvantage" and "triple jeopardy" have obstructed an understanding of multiple oppression because the equation one and one makes two, or one plus one plus one equals three does not work. Racism and disablism as two different forms of oppression cannot simply be added together to create a third' (Begum, 1994:31). Begum illustrates this argument:

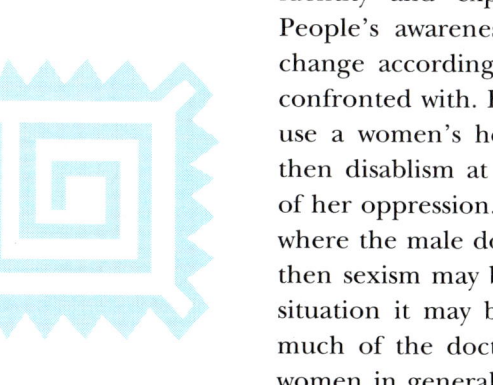

> In reality, most people are conscious of different aspects of their identity and experiences at different points in their lives. People's awareness and concern around particular issues can change according to the circumstances and situations they are confronted with. For example, if a white disabled woman cannot use a women's health centre because of steps at the entrance then disablism at that point may be the most significant aspect of her oppression. If she is forced to go to another health centre where the male doctor accuses her of being a 'hysterical woman' then sexism may be her greatest concern. However, in the latter situation it may be difficult for the woman to distinguish how much of the doctor's response is related to his perceptions of women in general, or how much it is related to an attitude that disabled people are asexual and consequently matters such as cervical smears, reproductive rights and breast screening are irrelevant to disabled women. (Begum, 1994:18)

Begum concludes 'our lives as Black Disabled people are comprised of many different facets and encompass a range of social divisions' (Begum, 1994:18). The experiences of black disabled people cannot be addressed by compartmentalising into neat discrete categories 'without understanding the influences, experiences and perceptions we might bring to a situation' (Begum, 1994:18). Begum proceeds to discuss Gloria Joseph (1981) who describes a situation where three black women are each facing a covered mirror. As the cover is raised the women see their reflections and confront the question 'Mirror, mirror on the wall, what is the greatest oppressor of us all?' The first woman responds by arguing that her Blackness is the central cause of her oppression and therefore white racism is the greatest oppression of all. The second woman claims that as a woman her life is controlled and dominated by men; consequently for her sexism is the greatest oppression of all. The third woman explains that it is not possible to give an immediate response because her gender, race and class are all sources of exploitation (Joseph and Lewis, 1981).

To summarise, seeing the lives of black disabled people as the sum of cumulative oppressions is simplistic. We need instead to develop an understanding that draws upon the concept of multiple and simultaneous oppression which sees disablism, racism and sexism impacting on the lives of black disabled people at any given time. Importantly, as Stuart (1992) points out, little of the existing research on black disabled people goes beyond conceptualising them in terms of 'double' or 'triple jeopardy'.

In the rest of this chapter we will firstly discuss issues relating to the extent of disability within the black community in Britain. Secondly, we describe the small number of key studies since the 1980 which have focused on the health and social care needs of black disabled people in order to establish what are the needs and how have they been met. Thirdly, we will attempt to illustrate black disabled people's experience of disability.

Demography

For the first time the 1991 Census included a question on limiting long term illness. Limiting long term illness is defined as 'Does the person have any long term illness, health problem or handicap which limits his/her daily activities or the work he/she can do?' The responses to the question are regarded by some as an indicator of the general level of health of the population[8] (Owen, 1994a:9). But the usefulness of the information yielded by the question is limited by the fact that all types of health problem are treated as being of equal severity. There is also uncertainty as to how people from black communities have interpreted this question (Charlton et al, 1994:22). Nevertheless it is worth using the information as a starting point.

The total number of residents in a household in Great Britain who were recorded as having such limiting long term illness was 6.67 million: 12.4 per cent. The proportion with limiting long term illness increased with age among both men and women: 30.2 per cent for those aged between 65 years of age to 62.2 per cent for those aged 85 plus.

Among the black communities the proportion of the population with limiting long term illness ranged from a low of 4.4 per cent for the Chinese to 11.2 per cent among the Black Caribbean group. Again, as in the white population, the incidence of limiting long term illness increased with age. It is important to recognise that:

> The age profiles of the population in these groups are not typical of those for the whole of Great Britain and these lower than average percentages reflect, to some degree, the extent to

which these ethnic minority populations are much younger than the white group. (Charlton et al, 1994:22).

However when rates were standardised for age they were lowest for Chinese men and women, highest for Bangladeshi men and Pakistani women. Women's rates tended to be higher than those for men, except for white, Bangladeshi and Chinese groups.

In terms of smaller scale or local studies, research reviewed by Atkin and Rollings (1993:10) does suggest that the incidence of disability among black people is higher than that for white people. They quote Farrah, 1986; Fenton, 1987; Moledina, 1988; and Ebrahim et al, 1991etc as evidence of higher levels of disability amongst black people compared to white people. However, Martin et al (1988) suggest that because of the differences in the age profiles of black and white communities - when standardised for age - the prevalence of disability amongst black people compared to white people is comparable.

Martin et al's (1988) analysis is partially supported by the recent Health and Lifestyles survey of black people by the Health Authority Education (1994). This found that when standardised for age there was little difference in current self-reported illness or disability between the UK population and the Afro-Caribbean and Indian population (27 per cent, 29 per cent and 26 per cent respectively). However, reported rates were higher amongst Pakistanis (30 per cent), and peaked at 36 per cent amongst Bangladeshis. The high rates of reported problems amongst both older Asian men and women (aged between 50 years and 74 years) were significantly higher than the UK population and Afro-Caribbean men and women.

To summarise, we are left with a picture which suggests that there are few instances where the prevalence of disability (or long term limiting illness) is lower in black communities than the white population when standardised for age. The national evidence for higher rates is unclear. However smaller scale or local studies do suggest higher rates (particularly for older people), but this may vary in terms of the constituent parts of the black communities. An unresolved issue with these studies remains in how to define disability.

Physical disability

As noted above, much of the available research which has focused on disability among black people has tended to concentrate on physical disability. This has been particularly so for black older people. An underlying theme has been that although black older people are younger compared to white older people, they do have considerable health and social care needs. For example, Afro-Caribbean and Asian pensioners in Birmingham reported more ill health and problems of physical mobility than their older white counterparts (Bhalla and Blakemore, 1981; Blakemore, 1983). Nine tenths of Afro-Caribbean older people in Leicester said that they had poor eyesight, a much higher proportion than would be expected amongst the population in general and, indeed, amongst old people from other ethnic groups (Farrah, 1986). Farrah also reported higher rates of stroke, hypertension and diabetes among black older people aged 55 and over compared with Hunt's (1978) survey of the elderly population as a whole (see chapter 4, page 57).

Furthermore, the research on physical disability highlights important inter-group variations. For example, a study by Derby Commission for Racial Equality of pensioners showed that the highest rate of reported illnesses occurred amongst Pakistani people (although they were not the most aged), but that there were disproportionately low rates amongst Indians (Derby CRE, nd). Indeed, these inter-group variations in relation to reported illnesses are also evidenced in the recent Health and Lifestyles survey by the Health Education Authority (1994) and the 1991 Census (Charlton et al, 1994).

Support for higher rates of disability amongst black communities comes from the link between health and social and economic circumstances. It has been argued that the physical and mental health of black people is adversely affected by the conditions they live in: poor living conditions, high unemployment, low income, institutional racism. Norman (1985) suggests the conditions in which black people live and work contribute to poor health and cites examples such as long hours of work in semi or unskilled manual work. Lewando-Hundt and Grant (1987) found that black people were more likely to be concentrated in manual and unskilled occupations than white people. These occupations, they argue, have higher incidences of health problems than other social groups (Townsend et al, 1988). A report from the Policy Studies Institute (Brown, 1984) describes the persistence of inequality for black people in respect of incomes, unemployment rates and poor housing. All three factors are related to ill health.

Sensory and/or learning disability

A small body of research is available which documents the health and social care needs of black people with sensory and/or learning disabilities (Lee, 1987; Cocking and Athwal, 1990; Baxter et al, 1990; Badat and Whall-Roberts, 1994; CIO, 1986). Lee (1987) focused on black families with one family member who had a mental handicap; Cocking and Athwal (1990) and Baxter (1990) focused on Asian families with children with learning disability; Badat and Whall-

Roberts (1994) focused on the needs of black deaf people; and the CIO (1986) study focused on a mixed sample of black people with physical/mobility disability, mental handicap, mental illness and sensory disability.

As in the case of physical disability among black older people, the prevalence of learning disability among black children appears to be higher than among white children (Baxter et al, 1990). Baxter and her colleagues summarise the evidence from several studies in 'northern mill towns'. They note:

> In Rochdale, for example, although only 5.5 per cent of the population in Rochdale was Asian, they made up 40 per cent of all the children attending the Development Therapy Unit and 35 per cent of the children receiving portage (Whitfield, 1988). A Manchester study revealed more of each type of severe disability (Akinsola and Fryers, 1986). In Oldham, Asian babies make up 18 per cent of the births, yet over a third of the under fives (double than the expected rate) have severe learning difficulties (BASW, 1987). Another study in Camberwell demonstrated that children with severe language impairment were significantly over-represented among children born to parents from the New Commonwealth (Wing, 1969). (Baxter et al, 1990:28)

Pathological explanations for this situation abound. Baxter et al (1990) note attempts to explain apparently higher prevalence of learning difficulties in some black communities with reference to two factors: a higher incidence of congenital rubella syndrome; and more frequent first cousin marriages. They suggest 'congenital rubella has been identified as two to three times higher in Asian than non Asian births in England and Wales (Miller et al, 1987)'. In reviewing this literature Baxter et al come out particularly strongly against first cousin marriages as an explanation because they suggest these conditions are rare enough to require '50 per cent consanguinity' (ie descended from the same ancestor) before they would lead to this level of learning disabilities. Baxter et al (1990:29) conclude that:

> It seems to be clear that congenital rubella syndrome and first cousin marriages cannot completely explain the relatively higher than expected proportion of black infants with learning difficulties.

It is likely, argue Baxter et al (1990:29), that 'most congenital abnormalities, including learning impairments, have causes present in the preconceptual period, at the time of conception and during the early weeks of pregnancy'. They then list poor housing, environmental pollution, inadequate and inappropriate education as other forms of material deprivation. As discussed in chapter 2, there is clear evidence that black communities have a higher risk of experiencing these forms of material deprivation.

To summarise, the evidence presented above does suggest that the incidence and prevalence of both physical and sensory and/or learning disabilities is higher amongst black communities. However, while congenital rubella syndrome and first cousin marriages may be in part the cause, there is evidence to show that this is unlikely to fully explain these levels of disability amongst black people. Socioeconomic factors appear to play a part and it is likely access to and delivery of services plays a part too.

The experience of disability

During the last decade attention has been drawn to the fact that the dual dimension of race and disability often makes the experiences of black disabled people and their carers different from those of the indigenous population (Begum, 1992). Evidence suggests that individual and institutional racism manifests itself in many aspects of the lives of black disabled people and their carers. Sometimes it is part and parcel of the everyday experiences of black non-disabled people, but at other times it is specific to the experience of disability and the factors associated with this. For example, in talking about sickle cell anaemia, Pamela Roberts explains:

> One of the most serious social issues that is affecting 'sicklers' at present is that . . . because sicklers usually have no . . . outward signs of painful crisis they are often considered to be stereotypes and labelled as malingerers and drug abusers (Roberts, 1991:3)

A study by the Confederation of Indian Organisations (CIO) in 1986 reported 'clear evidence of racial discrimination having affected the lives' of almost half of the sample interviewed. A number of them actually referred to the 'double discrimination' which was a reality of their daily existence:

> In some ways, yes, you have got a double problem with disabled people. Disabled people are second class citizens; when you are black or Asian you are third class. When I applied to a few companies and they found I was Asian and disabled that was it . . . When they see you are white they feel some sympathy, but once you are Asian or black that is it . . . It is the same thing as with the able-bodied people; the difference between the able white and the able Asian - the same thing applies; there's not much difference. (Interviewee, CIO, 1986:10)

Importantly, although the CIO sample was of working age (interviewees were aged between 17 and 54) only two were in employment: one man at Remploy and a woman in part-time work on sick leave and unsure of her return to work.

Begum (1992) notes 'racism and discrimination/harassment was a very real part of the lives of the people we interviewed' (Begum, 1992:65). The reality of this is poignantly highlighted in the responses of the disabled people interviewed: 'I sometimes wish I wasn't Asian so I didn't look the odd one out'. About half of the research sample reported that they had experienced racial harassment. This ranged from verbal abuse (experienced by 50 per cent of disabled people and 20 per cent of carers) to personal physical violence (14 per cent of the disabled people said they had experienced physical personal violence and seven per cent of carers). She quotes one respondent:

> Whilst sitting in a restaurant a white man walked in and screamed at me 'You blackie buy me breakfast'. I got scared and now I cannot go out because fear grips me and I keep feeling that something like this will happen again. (Disabled person, Begum, 1992:65)

> My child doesn't want to go to school anymore because she is frightened by the way children swear at her and attack her. (Carer, Begum, 1992:65)

Institutional racism has been cited as one of the barriers restricting opportunities and access to much needed resources:

> The myths may say that Britain's black and ethnic minority population is young, fit, transitory. It's not in need of community support services of this kind. Black communities have extensive family networks, they prefer to care for their own. But our research shows that black families with handicapped relatives are in as great, if not greater need of support from outside their immediate families as white. (Poonia and Ward, 1990:16)

In the CIO study over half of the sample lived with one or more parent, the rest either living alone (four) or with spouse (four), one in a sheltered residential home and one with a brother and her daughter. This, the authors state, was in excess of the norm for a group of this age. They suggest it is not because the Asian community look after their own but because the lack of awareness, availability and specific provision rendered no other choice. Cocking and Athwal (1990:12) conclude: 'The evidence from our survey therefore contradicts the commonly held view "Asians extended families look after their own"'.

Robina Shah, in her study looking at attitudes and stereotypes in terms of service provision to Asian families with a disabled child, writes:

> There is a consensus of thought among social workers that short term care is something quite abhorrent and unacceptable to the Asian community since it suggests that parents are incapable and incompetent to look after their own. This feeling of anti short term care was expressed by some of the parents interviewed, but this should not be taken to be representative of other Asian families . . . Such a negative response to short term care and fostering seems to reflect the lack of understanding Asian parents have about this particular service. Almost all of the parents in this study did not know what short term fostering involved. (Shah, 1986:2)

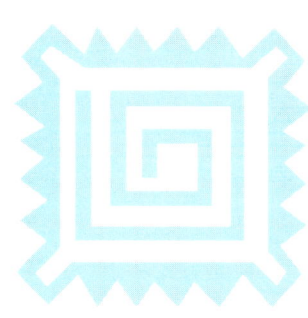

The fact that major surveys of the experience of disability persist in hardly mentioning the experience of black disabled people should not deter us from appreciating the messages that emerge from existing work. Racism, sexism and disablism intermingle to amplify the need for supportive social care. However these same factors sometimes mean that black disabled people and their carers get a less than adequate service.

Attitudes towards disability

It is frequently argued that black communities and in particular Asian communities view disability differently from the white community. A survey on the employment experiences of Asian disabled people notes:

> It has to be said that some of the related problems did seem to originate from within Asian communities themselves. Disability is sometimes seen as a 'curse' and this can cause the disabled person, particularly if a woman, to stay hidden away, or even worse to be hidden away. (CIO, 1986:10)

Such attitudes towards disability have been identified as one of the main factors which have deterred people from taking up services. For example, a report by GLAD (1987:4) of a study of disability among black people in three London boroughs points out that 'the general view in the social services departments was that the Asian communities regarded disability as a stigma and believed that a disabled person should be cared for within the whole family'.

Robina Shah specifically addresses the issue of attitudes in the Asian community. She notes that many social workers 'have various expectations of how Asian parents view their mentally/physically handicapped child'. These include stereotypes such as that Asian parents:

a reject their child immediately on finding out it has a disability/dis-abilities;

b encounter feelings of resentment by other members of their family;

c feel stigmatised by the family;

d see the birth of a disabled child as a punishment for sins or a test from God;

e promote feelings of inadequacy especially for the mother;

f express embarrassment;

g fail to see the necessity to prepare for the welfare of their child ie God will protect him/her;

h the Asian male is the dominant figure of the household and all communications should be made through him.

Shah argues that what this list completely dismisses is feelings of profound guilt, confusion and disbelief.

> But what parent, regardless of race, would not, she asks, have those very feelings? Such feelings are short-lived and parents begin to accept the situation and look for ways to help their child. (Shah, 1986:1)

Begum (1992:62) notes that, though 'there is evidence to suggest that attitudes towards disability in the Asian community are fairly negative', these have to be put into perspective. She found that:

- A lot of the ideas expressed were similar to those that prevail in the indigenous population.

- A lack of information and knowledge about disability leads people to formulate their ideas, opinions and expectations on the basis of myths and superstition.

- In many situations religious and cultural beliefs had become inter-twined and confused. For example, the notion that Muslims believe that disability is some form of punishment is likely to be based on cultural rather than religious grounds, because in Islam disability is not seen as a punishment but rather as a gift from God.

- As in any other community there was a lot of diversity in the atti-tudes and ideas which prevailed, some being more positive than others.

Clearly, the whole area of attitudes towards disability is complex. On the one hand, there is a body of literature pointing to a suggestion that disability is perceived in very negative terms, especially within the Asian community. On the other hand, writers are warning against the danger of stereotyping, without really looking for explanations or understanding some of the factors influencing people's thinking. However it is clear, points out Begum, that:

> Perhaps the only firm conclusion that can be drawn from the literature is that extreme caution needs to be exercised when trying to interpret the evidence. Whilst the difficulties associated with negative attitudes need to be acknowledged and responded to, great care also needs to be taken to ensure that the whole debate does not fall into the trap of blaming the 'victim'. (Begum, 1992:21)

It is important that service providers do not evade their responsibility by using negative attitudes towards disability and 'over protective families' as an excuse for the low take up of services and for ensuring an appropriate service which meets the specific needs of black disabled people and their carers.

Some studies suggest that for black people living in Britain disability has been given a low priority, because the process of living in Britain has meant there are a lot of other competing demands. Noel Perkins points out:

> It is only in the last twenty years that the indigenous population has come to accept that disabled people need access, equal opportunity and encouragement if they are to lead an active and purposeful life. It is not surprising then that disability does not yet have a high priority within the Afro-Caribbean community, most of whose time has been spent in tackling other priority areas such as housing. (GLAD, 1987:11)

Likewise, the CIO note that:

> A change in the Asian communities can come from the realisation that the disabled member is not a financial burden . . . To achieve this, what is needed is a campaign of educating the Asian communities regarding the services, welfare and employment available for disabled [people]. (CIO, 1987:17)

SCOPE, in their investigation of attitudes to disability, clearly demonstrate that negative attitudes are probably universal (Lamb and Lazelle, 1994). The studies reviewed here suggest that to see the struggle of black disabled people with other black people as symptomatic of a community specific attitude to disability is probably wrong.

Knowledge and use of services

A significant finding by the studies which have focused on black disabled people is the lack of knowledge about social and health services and their use. As the other chapters in this review have noted, this is a theme constantly repeated in an examination of incidence, prevalence and characteristics of social care needs of black people.

Badat and Whall-Roberts (1994) found that many Asian deaf people 'have almost no knowledge of services provided by local authorities or other agencies. A significant number of Asian deaf people are not receiving the services that could enable them to enjoy equality of opportunity' (Badat and Whall-Roberts, 1994:10). They further noted that links between local authorities in West Yorkshire and Asian community groups, and groups for Asian deaf people in particular, were patchy. The local authority was often not in touch with relevant community groups for Asian people, and there was consequently little consultation over needs and services. Similarly, a study by the Asian Disability Advisory Project Team (ADAPT) found that many of the Asian families interviewed had no knowledge of the services available (ADAPT, 1993). Begum (1992) comments on take up of services in her study of Asian disabled people and their carers in Waltham Forrest: 'The number of people using services was so small that it was not worth doing a comparison between carers and people with disabilities' (Begum, 1992:81). (The main services used over the previous year, predominantly by carers, were respite care and day nurseries.)

Echoing this point, other studies have shown that those who care for black disabled people also know very little of services available and consequently under use them (see chapter 7, page 109). For example, Cocking and Athwal (1990:12) note: 'There was a considerable lack of knowledge about local services for people with learning difficulties'. For example, 23 people were incontinent yet only six of their families knew about the incontinence laundry scheme.

Language barriers and lack of accessible information have been identified as one of the biggest obstacles faced by black disabled people and their carers in getting knowledge about services. A conference report on Asians and disabilities points out that:

> Asian people's experiences of disabilities are essentially different from other people with disabilities because of language difficulties and institutional racism. There appears to be a severe lack of accessible information regarding available services, such as employment, education, training, recreation, grants and allowances for disabled people. (CIO, 1987:7)

The issue is discussed by other studies: Begum (1992) for example found that access to information in an appropriate form was one of the main factors preventing black disabled people and carers from taking up services in the London Borough of Waltham Forrest. Cocking and Athwal (1990) noted that many of the Asian parents of children with learning difficulties in their sample had little contact with school teachers or day centre staff. They conclude:

> While the same is true to some extent of the UK European families in the sample, the problem was exacerbated for the Asian families by language difficulties. (Cocking and Athwal, 1990:12)

Communication and access to information is not a problem restricted to those who do not speak English, but presents difficulties for other black people too. Noel Perkins found that many of the Afro-Caribbean disabled people could not understand the complex jargon of the claims procedure unless someone with patience and understanding explained it to them. He notes:

> People should be told not only what services are available but also the extent of the powers of social services departments, because some of the questions they were asked during assessment for services were perceived as unnecessary and too personal. (GLAD, 1987:12)

Therefore evidence that social services departments have begun to translate material as well as provide interpreters is a sign of progress; but this should take place in the context of ensuring that communication is improved with all black communities.

Insensitive or inappropriate services

Beyond lack of information and communication barriers, it also is likely that many of the services currently available tend to be insensitive or inappropriate to the specific needs of black people. For example, the ADAPT study found that where services had been used these had been rejected because they were deemed inappropriate to their specific needs. This was illustrated by the following case:

> During an interview with a 24 year old disabled person the interviewer was told about his father. He was 70 years old and after being paralysed in an accident wore incontinence pads. His daughter-in-law had changed his pads for two years. She said she found it humiliating as for both of them it was a degrading experience. Finally a worker was sent to help with the task of changing the incontinence pads. This new worker was an Asian woman. The family found this just as embarrassing and declined

the use of the service after two days. The family asked why a male worker could not have been sent. (ADAPT, 1993:16)

An often cited barrier to providing a service which is not only sensitive and appropriate but specific to individual's needs is a lack of knowledge amongst care providers of what those needs are and the commitment to change. Badat and Whall-Roberts (1994) found that professionals (including social workers, health visitors and GPs) who came into contact with deaf people from black communities were often unaware of the cultural and religious implications of their advice. They conclude that 'This can mean that they give inappropriate or unhelpful advice' (Badat and Whall-Roberts, 1994:20). GLAD (1987) similarly found that though statutory providers had some knowledge of the kinds of needs amongst Asian disabled people, they were not aware of their specific needs. This they noted was evident in the low uptake of services. The lack of ethnic record keeping and monitoring further accentuated the problem and appeared to contribute to statutory bodies being unable to plan provision adequately.

The ADAPT study (1993) further recorded that, with a couple of notable exceptions, the majority of services are taken up by only a small percentage of Asian users. Whilst a number of service providers had taken steps to make their services more accessible to Asian people, others had not taken any. This was often in the face of knowledge that the available service was not being used.

A recent study of care management in three local authorities by Begum (1995) found that there were few alternatives open to black people if a care package which included specific services turned out to be inappropriate. For example, one elderly Asian man required a Muslim man to provide personal care, but despite extensive attempts to find an appropriate person, a Sikh man was recruited to provide the support. Begum notes that 'the lack of appropriate alternative services meant that some black users were left in somewhat difficult and compromising situations' (Begum, 1995:3). One black physically disabled man had already spent 12 years in a residential home where he was the only black user, and a substantial distance away from his family. He had managed to negotiate (with some difficulty) the provision of food appropriate to his needs, but his over-riding requirement was to live near his family with 14 hours of support. The user did not seem to think his care package had been reviewed since the implementation of care management, but he was somewhat sceptical about what care management could offer him, as he was not aware of any independent living services in the area where his family lived.

Conclusion

In conclusion, what the exact incidence and prevalence of disability amongst black people is remains the subject of debate. What is clear is that the level of disability amongst black people is likely to be either at the same rate and certainly no less than that in the white population. The studies reviewed here demonstrate the existence of disability amongst black communities and the extent of their needs. The studies reviewed further show that access to and knowledge of services is low amongst both black disabled people and their carers.

The experience of disability is different for black disabled people than for their white counterparts. Black disabled people have to contend with discrimination and disadvantage associated with their disability and as a result of racism. However, care must be taken with viewing black disabled people's lives in terms of competing or cumulative oppressions. The reality is likely to see different situations bringing different oppressions to prominence, as well as highlighting the importance of past experiences of individuals.

Finally, if higher rates of disability are found (as has been suggested by some work on learning disability) we need to be careful not to immediately focus on pathological explanations such as first cousin marriages. The impact of socio-economic factors and issues relating to access to and delivery of services has been demonstrated as playing a part in the incidence of these disabilities in white people, and they are likely to play a part in terms of black communities also.

7

Carers

Summary

The small number of studies on informal care within black communities show that the mainstay of this care are predominantly women. Furthermore that caring is not a new phenomenon, with many of these women having been principle carers for some years. Also that the needs of black carers are numerous ranging from education on health, diet and care, to support with caring. Importantly, just as is the case for some white carers, carers in black communities appear to be unsupported and isolated. This is often exacerbated by communication difficulties and the lack of sensitive and appropriate services. Service provision continues to remain ethnocentric, geared to meeting the needs of the white majority. Further, there is evidence to show that black carers are often more severely affected by the problems of poverty and bad housing.

Studies also explode the myth of 'black people looking after their own'. It appears we confuse the higher proportion of multi-generational households in black communities as evidence of the existence of caring relationships. Additionally, there is evidence that the extended network of family support is not so readily achievable in England because of migration patterns which have tended to divide families. Finally, studies also suggest that simply living in a large family does not always mean that support is available and that the needs of those being cared for and those caring are adequately met.

There is little work on informal care which examines the experience of caring by black people (Twigg, 1992). Mainstream research, like mainstream service provision, has remained largely ethnocentric in that this has paid little attention to examining the needs of black carers and those that they care for (see Parker and Lawton, 1994). The exclusion of black carers from mainstream research has added to the invisibility of black carers, their specific need requirements and of those that they care for. Evandrou (1994) in her recent review of studies on black older people noted that this continues to be the failing of research.

Though the studies considered here are small (maximum sample size 50) and local, they nevertheless highlight that just as in the white community, carers in black communities are unsupported and isolated. The mainstay of day care in the main tend to be women. The lack of support for and isolation of black carers is particularly exacerbated by the lack of appropriate service provision, greater poverty, bad housing and racism.

This chapter will describe the key studies on informal care and black communities since the 1980s to the present in order to establish whether needs exist, and if they do how they have been met by service providers. In addition, we will examine issues relating to demography and the socio-economic circumstances of black carers; and consider the existence of the extended family network and its ability to meet the needs of carers and those cared for. Inevitably in this report there is some repetition when we discuss carers in the same contexts as the other chapters on black elders and disability.

Demography

The General Household Survey estimated that 6.7 million people care for sick, elderly or disabled people, within the same household (Green, 1988). According to the British Medical Association one in seven adults provides regular care to a friend, neighbour or close relative, with 1.7 million people heavily involved in hands-on caring (Carrington, 1995).

These statistics, however, do not give any information about the number and circumstances of carers who are black. From the evidence discussed in chapter 4 it is apparent that while the percentage of black elders is lower than for the white community, they may be more likely to be ill or frail. Evidence presented in chapter 6 suggests that there may also be higher rates of impairment or disability. While both chapters suggest we need to be cautious about the ability (or willingness) of black families to care for black elders or black disabled people, there is no evidence to suggest that there are fewer people who actually care than is the case for white people. It seems reasonable to suggest that once we account for the differing make up of black and white communities (fewer black older people for example) we are likely to find proportionately similar or possibly higher numbers of black carers.

Carers' needs

From the late 1980s a number of studies have concentrated primarily on the experiences of caring by black carers. These studies have focused on exploring the needs of carers and those they care for. Further, these studies have explored whether service provision has been able to meet those needs.

For example, a study by McCalman (1990) of 34 carers from three minority ethnic communities - Afro-Caribbean, Asian and Vietnamese/Chinese - living in the London Borough of Southwark found that all the carers looked after a close relative: just over half cared for a parent, step parent or parent-in law, one third cared for a spouse, and just over an eighth cared for grandparents. Twenty-one carers were female (62 per cent of all those interviewed) and 13 carers were men (38 per cent). In exploring the tasks undertaken by black carers McCalman found that 21 carers undertook some kind of personal care, and 24 provided physical help such as lifting or help with walking. All the carers reported substantial time spent in caring activities: 25 carers, for example, spent over 11 hours per day caring for older relatives. Carers also reported that they had spent a considerable amount of their lives caring: five had been caring for 11 years and 28 for over two years. Further, a high proportion lived with those cared for (77 per cent), with the remainder living on their own.

This study further highlighted that black carer's needs were numerous and varied. These included education on health, diet, and caring as well as help with day-to-day life in a predominantly white society. Other needs included the breakdown of language barriers, access to information and services, physical help with caring, relief care for their elderly relatives, links with social services, health and volunteer services, adequate housing, emergency help line and adequate financial means. The needs of elderly relatives varied according to their disabilities and position within their families. For example, those whose physical needs were being met by their carers, expressed the need for faculties they had lost such as seeing or walking. Those who lived alone and had to look after themselves when their carers were absent asked to be near their carers or wanted them to fulfil more of their physical needs. McCalman concludes that although the sample size was small:

> If there were any notions that caring was not happening in minority communities, or that extended families within them made caring easier, this report provides strong evidence to the contrary. Minority ethnic carers are caring in the same way as white carers. (McCalman, 1990:72)

Lee (1987) in a sample study of 26 black carers caring for 'mentally handicapped' people (Afro-Caribbean and Asian) found again that the mainstay of care were women caring for a close relative (23 were parents, two grandparents and one a sibling). The study highlighted that the extended family for the majority of carers was the only source of support. Some support was being received from voluntary organisations and religious bodies, although this was by no means widespread. Valuable support noted by white carers in the first stage of the study provided by neighbours was not available to black carers caring for a mentally handicapped person. The needs of carers in relation to using health and social services were reluctantly voiced. The reason for this was not because these black carers had no needs of their own or that their needs were being met, but more because existing provision was seen as inappropriate and therefore unacceptable. For example, 47 out of the 64 people being cared for had problems with self care; 38 had serious behaviour problems making their management difficult; and 13 had severe to moderate incontinence problems. Since these numbers above relate to different families not the same families:

> The cumulative picture means that half of the families in the sample are dealing either with serious behaviour difficulties or with a severe problem of incontinence. (Lee, 1987:14)

Cameron et al (1988) in a study of black older women with disability and black women who were carers found that as in the white community women were the mainstay of care provided to black older people who were frail or disabled. For example, out of the 25 carers participating in the study 20 were women. The study further highlights the lack of support and isolation experienced by black carers. Cameron et al quote the case of one respondent:

> A 66 year old Asian widow, Mrs Sharma, who came from Africa in the 1960s was severely disabled since a stroke in 1985. She lived with her son, daughter-in-law, who was her main carer, and two granddaughters. She was very dependent, day and night, needed help with toileting and feeding and had difficulty speaking. Her daughter-in-law never left her except when she had relief care every two months. Even then her daughter-in-law visited daily and took in her main meal. Mrs Sharma's daughter-in-law had a little English and said she felt tied to the house: 'Sometimes I am very tired'. Despite help from services, her own life was severely restricted by her mother-in-law's ill health. (Cameron et al, 1988:24)

Another disadvantage, note Cameron et al, that:

> black women faced in their role as carers was physical isolation: some were restricted to their houses through fear of an 'alien' outside world where their own norms, values and social skills were often regarded as inappropriate, their behaviours in danger of misrepresentation or where they were confronted by many subtle expressions of racism. (Cameron et al, 1988:22)

This reduced the possibility of chance encounters which, argue Cameron et al:

for old white women and their carers in our study had sometimes proved to be the first step in getting help from other agencies, statutory or voluntary; old black women were 'invisible' as were the disabled people they cared for. (Cameron et al, 1988:22)

In Cameron et al's work it appears that the responsibility of caring often began very early in life. For example, the study showed that girls from Asian families were the ones who were required to act as interpreters for their disabled grandparents, sometimes missing school and having to cope with 'adult' problems, concerns and situations in their interpreting role. Cameron et al conclude that although black carers share many of the disadvantages that affect white carers, black carers face a further disadvantage 'because of the colour of their skin. As carers or cared for they are largely invisible to the wider society' (Cameron et al, 1988:32). Because of this service provision has continued to remain ethnocentric and discriminatory, 'geared to the white majority and makes little or no provision for minorities' (Cameron et al, 1988:33).

To summarise, it is clear from the small number of studies on informal care within the black community that the mainstay of this care are women. Furthermore, that caring is not a new phenomenon: for example there is evidence to show that many of the carers have been caring up to 11 years. In addition the studies suggest that the needs of black carers are numerous, ranging from education on health, diet and care, to support for and information on caring. Importantly, just as is the case for some white carers, carers in black communities are unsupported and isolated. This appears to be compounded by both discrimination and the continuation of service provision geared towards meeting the needs of the white majority.

Poverty, housing and employment

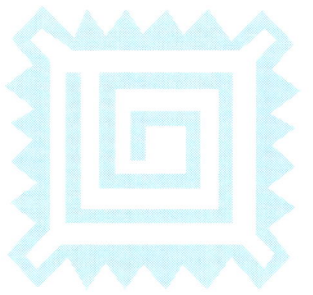

Though the experience of black carers was similar to white carers there is some evidence that for black carers the burden of care was often greater, both socially and financially. Many of the studies on informal care within black communities show that black carers often had more severe problems of poverty, bad housing and racism; with Cocking and Athwal (1990), for example, finding a high level of unemployment among the families in their study.

Cameron et al (1988) note 'another disadvantage was that black carers,' particularly women, 'were likely to have limited access to financial resources'. This was due to many of the women carers in the study being recent arrivals in Britain with little or no money, and because of low paid working and minimal pension rights. The low level of pensions rights within the black communities is well documented amongst the research on black older people (see chapter 4 page 62).

McCalman (1990) reports that the problems of poor heating, bad housing, the reality of racial attacks and lack of money for many of the black carers were more immediate and pressing. For example, she found that of the eight Asian carers, five lived in council dwellings. One carer lived in rented accommodation owned by a housing association, two in owner-occupied terraced houses, and one in a flat. Three carers living on the same estate were found to be living in very poor and inadequate housing. The approach to the flats was dirty, rooms were cold and unattractive and there were no lifts. Two of the three carers living there felt that a change in accommodation was their prime concern, and she notes that 'in conversation, this seemed to take precedence over their caring role' (McCalman, 1990:47).

McCalman also found that most often carers supported the relatives cared for financially, from either earnings or family benefits received. For example, she found that all Asian carers and nine of the Afro-Caribbean carers supported their elderly relatives. Furthermore, many of the black carers participating in the study reported that they found it financially difficult to provide the care their elderly relatives needed.

In similar fashion to McCalman, Gunaratnum (1990) argues that issues like racial harassment, bad housing, and the lack of financial assistance are as much carers' issues for black carers as respite care or sitting services. She notes that 'the most important point for the carers was that these issues cannot be separated from their caring' (Gunaratnum, 1990: no page numbers). For example, for one carer in the study his poor housing conditions were more of a pressure and indeed added pressure to his caring. Another carer was more immediately concerned to protect herself and her husband from racial harassment. She warns that restricting 'real carers' issues to just the caring situation and relationship' means whole parts of black carers' experiences will go unaddressed (Gunaratnum, 1990: no page numbers).

In summary, there is some evidence to show that black carers are often more severely affected by the problems of poverty, bad housing and racism. These concerns are part and parcel of their daily life and cannot be isolated from their role of caring.

Extended family network

The idea that black people 'look after their own' is particularly common in relation to informal care. The commitment of black families to care for older and disabled relatives is assumed to be greater than that of white people, to the extent that service provision thinks it need not concern itself with the needs of black people. This appears to be so notwithstanding research which draws attention to the fact that the supportive extended family is possibly a myth. 'Perhaps the most revealing finding of this research' concluded Baxter 'is the shattering of these assumptions' (Baxter, 1989:8). Cocking and Athwal similarly concluded in their study of Asian carers that 'the evidence from our survey . . . contradicts the commonly held view that Asian extended families look after their own'. (Cocking and Athwal, 1990:12)

Evidence from the Labour Force Survey suggests almost a third of all black people live in small family households (one or two persons aged 16 or above and one or two persons under 16 according to the 1988/90 Survey). Although the extended family is common among Asian families, there is still a significant proportion who live alone, particularly those with few relatives in this country (see Atkin et al, 1989; Cameron et al, 1988; Baxter, 1989; McCalman, 1990). It appears that the traditional pattern in many Asian communities of the responsibility of care being shared among a network of family members is not so readily achievable in Great Britain. Firstly, because migration in itself has tended to divide families. Baxter (1989:7) notes that 'immigration laws and procedures posed added strain on some families' caring for people with cancer. She quotes one respondent:

> If only it was easier for relatives to come over from Pakistan. I would get my niece to come over and help, but it is so difficult nowadays to come over even as visitors so we have to struggle on. (Baxter, 1989:7)

Secondly, changes in family and household structure as well as the geographical dispersal of kin make it increasingly difficult for Asian family life to continue around the extended kinship network. For example, McCalman (1990) noted that Asian carers had an alarmingly high degree of isolation. This, she states, was because there was 'very little family help except from their own children. Many had no other family members nearby' (McCalman, 1990:66). Furthermore, as in the white community, the caring, even when a family network was available, was still seen as the responsibility of the main carer (see McCalman, 1990; Cocking and Athwal, 1990). McCalman, for example, found that help from other family members by Afro-Caribbean carers was constrained to close relatives: husband, wife, children and sometimes siblings. Other family members such as aunts, uncles, cousins, nephews and nieces sometimes visited but were not directly involved in caring. She notes that in the case of Asian carers they all said they received help from other family members. This included, again, close relatives such as carers' children and siblings.

Cameron et al similarly note:

> With the changes in family structure, household composition and geographical dispersal of close and extended kin, black women carers were sometimes left to care for someone more or less on their own, without family support. The traditional pattern of care 'back home' which would involve sharing responsibilities and duties amongst a network of family members was not so readily available. For Asian women the new experience of caring for a disabled person, which typifies the 'individualised' response to disability in western society, was often an alien and unanticipated one. (Cameron et al, 1988:22)

Living in a large family does not necessarily mean that service support is not needed or that all the needs of those caring and cared for are adequately being met. It could be that people are resigned to their situation because of the lack of knowledge about service provision and access. Barker (1984), for example, in a study of black older people in London and Manchester noted that by contrast to white older people and Afro-Caribbean older people, Asian older people were more likely to live with large households. He found that many of the old men in the study, particularly those who had joined their children over the last 15 years, felt of little value to the household where young relatives were busy and left them feeling lonely during large parts of the day. Turnbull (1985) similarly notes that the 'maintenance of a traditional extended family pattern for the majority may hide the most vulnerable minority'. Furthermore, she adds that 'even within the extended family setting there was often conflict and loneliness' (Turnbull, 1985:20). And a recent study suggests that an expressed need for respite services was twice as high for Asian families as for white families (Robinson and Stalker, 1992).

To summarise, we appear to assume the higher proportion of multi-generational households in black communities is evidence of the existence of caring relationships. Furthermore, there is evidence that black carers face similar situations to those of their white counterparts. For example the burden of care, as in the white community, often falls on one principal carer. Support from other family members is limited to close relatives such as spouse, siblings and children, again similar to white carers. Additionally, there is evidence that the extended network of family support is not so readily achievable in Great Britain because of migration patterns which have tended to divide families. Finally, simply living in a large family does not always mean that support is not needed and that the needs of those being cared for and those caring are adequately met.

Knowledge and use of services

A common theme amongst all the studies looking at informal care within the black community is the lack of knowledge about service provision and under use of available services. For example, a study by Cocking and Athwal (1990) looking at Asian carers with children with learning difficulties found that very few carers knew what services were available and how to access them: they found 23 people in the study were incontinent, yet only six carers knew about the incontinence laundry scheme. Furthermore, they found that almost half did not know about respite care, and only a third of the sample used this service. Where services were being accessed, it appeared to be because of chance rather than design. Cocking and Athwal quote the case of one respondent:

> Ms Sandhu had met another parent at the hospital who had told her about the benefit. She then claimed it - successfully - but could have claimed it nine years earlier. She was also able to claim Invalid Care Allowance, which she had previously been unaware of, as a result of the interview. (Cocking and Athwal, 1990:12)

Similarly Baxter (1989), in a study looking at support and information needs of people with cancer and their carers, found that though attitudes and beliefs did not differ widely from the majority communities in relation to cancer, what was interesting was the lack of knowledge of services, especially among non-English speaking and older people. She notes that the 'absence of translated materials in relevant languages and their dissemination often meant that black carers did not know about the existence of services and where to go to get them' (Baxter, 1989:5). She quotes one respondent:

> We were not aware that mother could get help. Perhaps if she knew, she would not have stayed on at work so long. Her financial situation was difficult at the time and that is why she continued working and suffering. (Baxter, 1989:7)

McCalman (1990) also found that although take up and awareness of services was low among all carers, among black carers this was even lower. This was particularly the case for such services as holiday breaks and services relating to personal care and community nursing. Language was a big barrier for many carers: for example, of all the services available to give carers a break only 21 per cent used a social services day centre, the majority tending to take advantage of community day centres and luncheon clubs. Services providing longer breaks such as council run holidays for older people and older people with disability were not generally used or heard of. Of the services provided in the home, home help was the most known, though this was limited to elderly carers. In terms of use of services, aids and adaptation services were used by 15 per cent of the elderly relatives; meals on wheels by only three per cent. There were instances where people knew of services like meals on wheels but did not use them because they were unhappy with it.

Cole (1990) found that where people were using services they often had limited knowledge of the scope of the service being used. For example, many of the respondents were not sure what the duties of a home care worker were. This meant that in some cases home care workers took advantage of their ignorance. For example, she found that home care workers, when asked, told black clients that they were not allowed to do some jobs.

Chiu (1989) in a study of informal care among a sample of Chinese older people found that 90 per cent of the Chinese older people interviewed had not received any help from social workers, home help, community nurses or meals on wheels, despite the fact that needs were apparent. For example, the research revealed a high level of need for care among Chinese older people: 45 per cent of the respondents said bathing was difficult to do alone, another 40 per cent had difficulty in putting on footwear, 50 per cent said they had difficulty going to the toilet. The main reason for not using services was that though services were available they were not accessible in practice. Some Chinese older people, particularly those who were isolated and unattached to any service agency, were not aware of the existence of such services. Those that had heard of them did not know enough to enable or encourage them to apply. Another reason for the under use was that much of what was available was often regarded by Chinese older people as inappropriate. Meals on wheels, for example: more than 40 per cent of the Chinese older people interviewed in the research indicated that the meals provided did not suit a Chinese diet.

In summary, much of the evidence discussed so far shows that knowledge and use of services is lower amongst black communities. This is often exacerbated by communication difficulties.

Barriers

Even if black carers know about services there is evidence to show that these are rejected because what is on offer is either inappropriate, inadequate and not flexible enough to meet individual needs.

Cocking and Athwal (1990) found that services were often rejected because they were inappropriate. They quote one respondent:

> Mr and Mrs Rashid, in their 60s and caring for their adult daughter who was seriously ill, had turned down respite care in the past because they were told it was only available in blocks of one or two weeks. They wanted occasional nights so that they could attend weddings and funerals. (Cocking and Athwal, 1990:12)

Cocking and Athwal argue that services need:

> to be more flexible, and to be offered not just once but several times in accordance with people's needs changing over time. (Cocking and Athwal, 1990:12)

They further noted that although all but two people with learning difficulties were at either school, nursery or attending social services day care, there was often very little contact between carers and service providers. Cocking and Athwal argue that while the same is true to some extent of the UK European families in the sample, the problem was exacerbated for the Asian families by language difficulties. They quote one respondent:

> Mr and Mrs Mishra never attended reviews at their daughter's day centre. In fact they had never visited there, and their only contact was by phone. Mr Mishra's command of English was not good; consequently he did not understand everything that was said. The family would have liked regular reports on Sushma's progress, or to have had some assistance via an interpreter, in understanding reviews. (Cocking and Athwal, 1990:12)

Cocking and Athwal conclude that this could have been easily rectified by providing an interpreter who would be available to make home visits with day centre staff and be present at review days.

Baxter (1989) notes that the lack of flexibility by service providers meant that black carers and those that they cared for were not given the necessary assistance which would have made their work easier and helped their relatives to develop independence. She quotes one respondent:

It tore me apart to see my mother struggle up the stairs, because due to her religious convictions she refused to use the commode (as a muslim you are supposed to wash yourself after using the toilet). I applied to the Social Security for a chair lift and I was told because she was over 60 she did not qualify for it. They could not understand the importance of her religion. (Baxter, 1989:7)

Lee (1987) concludes from his study that:

What emerges here is that carers are having to make do with an unsatisfactory situation rather than having the opportunity to choose a culturally appropriate diet for their dependants. (Lee, 1987:7)

The lack of appropriate service which is accessible to all groups is further demonstrated by Cole (1990). When questioned on respite care, out of all the respondents three were in receipt of respite care, ten were unaware of what the term 'respite care' meant, seven had a vague idea of what respite care involved. However, all were prepared to accept respite care depending on:

- The ethnic sensitivity of services available.

- Accessibility of service by the client.

- Accessibility in terms of distance and quality of services.

Meals on wheels were considered to be inappropriate to black dietary needs. When questioned on what more could be provided, eight said they were unaware of what current or additional services were available, therefore were not able to answer. The remainder of the sample recommended the following: increase in help, and information on available services.

Cole's study found that services were planned with little consultation with the black communities and black carers. Cole believes this was one reason why services remained inappropriate and inflexible. Further, that often the needs of black carers were not considered in assessment. Assessments tended to focus only on the needs of the person being cared for. When questioned as to whether work, personal and family commitments were taken into account, 50 per cent said they were not; two were unable to answer the question. The reasons given by seven carers for the assessor's inability to be sensitive were:

- Carers were not informed by assessors of available services relevant to their needs.

- Insensitivity as evidenced by length of allocated time of worker which did not allow for in-depth assessment of needs.

- Told by assessor that family should be doing more to help and thereby made the family feel guilty.

Those who delivered services also showed little awareness of the needs of black clients. For example, the majority said that black clients had the same needs as white clients. Cole noted that the answers given are a clear indication of attitudes and working practices of home care workers towards black clients. She concludes:

> The views reflect a Colour Blind Approach . . . People holding this position negate black people's specific experience of racism both in services and the wider community. (Cole, 1990:25)

Gunaratnum (1990) argues that services need to be imaginative and flexible in order to meet the specific needs of black carers. Such an approach can improve services to all, not just to black carers. In a study of Asian carers she found that 'Asian carers' as a group do not exist. The experiences of the carers differed according to who they were and where they lived. The needs of Bengali carers in Tower Hamlets, for example, were different to the needs of Punjabi carers in Derby. In support of this she found that all the carers in Tower Hamlets lived in council housing and most of them did not read or write. In such a situation translated information made little difference to those who could not read nor had access to friends/families who could. This left many Asian carers in the study feeling they rather than the services were the problem. As one carer said:

> If only I knew how to read and write, I would know where to go, what to do and whom I should see. I wouldn't have all these problems. (Gunaratnum, 1990: no page numbers)

Gunaratnum argues that illiteracy is obviously an issue that can affect all carers, yet little progress appears to have been made in exploring different ways of information giving. At its most basic, lack of appropriate information is disenfranchising carers from their right to services. As one carer said:

> These days you have to fight for your rights, but I don't know what my rights are. (Gunaratnum, 1990: no page numbers)

The most useful examples of support given to Asian carers are those which are sufficiently flexible to enable carers to define their own needs, from their own experiences. In Camden, for example, when it was found that a carer's group would not be appropriate, a system of volunteer visiting to carers was initiated by an Asian community worker in consultation with the carers.

The ethos of flexibility and creativeness is also echoed by McCalman (1990) and Cocking and Athwal (1990). Cocking and Athwal noted:

> It is clear that a number of families need information disseminated in a form other than the written word, for example by making video and audio cassettes, in addition to translating leaflets. (Cocking and Athwal, 1990:13)

A recent study by Walker and Ahmad (1994) concludes that the statutory services are ill equipped to meet the needs of black older people and their carers. Though community care opens up possibilities, these can only be realised if it is recognised how problematic the stereotypical expectation is, the extent of the pressures on black carers and the limitation of the black voluntary sector.

In summary, evidence suggests that service provision continues to remain ethnocentric, geared to meeting the needs of the white majority. Until service providers recognise the importance of services to cater for all needs, black carers will continue to be marginalised and remain invisible.

Conclusion

While the notion of the extended family raises the possibility of a range of carers, evidence shows that just as in the white community carers in the black community are unsupported and isolated. However, the lack of knowledge with regard to services, both for carers and those cared for, and the particular barriers to access and delivery have meant that for black carers the burden of caring is higher than for the white carers. This has been exacerbated by the higher levels of poverty and bad housing, and a service provision geared to meeting only the needs of the white majority.

Summary and Conclusion

All too often those attempting to promote the rights of Britain's black communities have resorted to presenting these communities as passive victims of an aggressive state. This has sometimes led to a failure to acknowledge the positive contribution that some agencies and individuals have made (and are continuing to make) in the provision of social care, as well as ignoring the role played by black communities themselves. In then attempting to discuss the incidence, prevalence and characteristics of social care needs, there is the possibility of presenting a one-dimensional picture because the main concern is to identify those in need and what their needs are. This may further contribute to the 'victimology'[9] of black communities. Therefore it must be remembered that Britain's black communities do survive and prosper. However, they do have social care needs and this review attempts to identify these.

Demography

In terms of demography there is clear evidence that there are few areas of Britain where black communities do not have a presence. This is true both in terms of local authority districts but also at ward level. However, for the most part black communities continue to live in areas with higher than average numbers of black people. Once again this is true at the local authority district level, and is particularly so at the ward level. Furthermore, in a number of wards black communities constitute almost half of the local population and in some cases they constitute the ethnic majority group.

These conclusions emphasise the need to ensure that the provision of appropriate services to black communities is on the agenda of all social care providers, as none can claim that this is not a 'problem' for them. More importantly they suggest that for some social work teams or frontline service providers a significant number of the potential client group will be from black communities. They also suggest the need to have detailed knowledge of local populations, because the level of spatial concentration is such that neighbouring wards and districts can have dramatically different populations. Finally, our discussions suggest that the potential for isolation - where black communities are a small fraction of the size of the white population - is very real.

Other demographic characteristics highlighted are that black communities are younger then their white counterparts, with 33 per

cent of 'ethnic minorities' under 15 as opposed to 19 per cent of
white people. On the other end of the scale, over 39 per cent of white
people are over the age of 45 as opposed to over 18 per cent of
'ethnic minorities'. The significant number of children in black
communities is now being accompanied by a small but growing number of black people of pensionable age and over. However, for the
most part women do not outnumber men in the over 60 black
population as they do in white communities.

This review also shows that black communities have larger households
than their white counterparts. This is partially explained by the above
average number of households that have three or more adults (a
possible indicator of the existence of extended families). However,
the most important factor appears to be the above average number of
children in ethnic minority households/family units.

Although the analysis of household structure emphasises the
prevalence of families with children under the age of 16, it also shows
the existence of pensioner households. No 'ethnic minority group'
has the same percentage of pensioner households or lone pensioner
households as white communities do. However, they do appear to
exist in most communities and most often for black Caribbeans,
probably reflecting their earlier arrival to this country.

When it is possible to look at the change in the size of the black
communities between 1981 and 1991, it is clear that they have grown.
The rate of growth in the constituent parts of black communities varies, with the Bangladeshi community growing the most in percentage
terms and Pakistanis in actual numbers. Much of this growth is
explained by natural growth (more births then deaths) rather than
net migration (more people coming than leaving Great Britain),
although this plays a significant part in the growth of Bangladeshis.
Finally, although we reviewed some evidence that suggests that the
size of the Caribbean community is declining, we need to be cautious
as to how much this reflects a change in the size of the community as
opposed to a change in the categories this community has chosen to
use in the 1991 Census.

We examined social and economic circumstances focusing on the
work of David Owen and the Department of Environment (Robson et
al, 1995 and Coombes et al, 1995). Neither Owen nor the DOE report
authors suggest that their analysis of deprivation (or affluence) means
that black communities are experiencing deprivation. However, both
Owen and the DOE are clear that these communities live in areas
where deprivation is more pronounced. Black communities are at
greater risk of experiencing unemployment, and this is more likely to

be long term; overcrowding, as well as children living in unsuitable accommodation (even though owner occupation is high amongst groups such as Pakistanis); and persons or households living on income support. Importantly for our review, this evidence suggests that black communities are at greater risk of experiencing some of the stresses so often associated with people who need the services of social care agencies.

Children and families

There can be little doubt that black children need to be protected, just as white children do. Similarly they need to have their welfare promoted. While the development of preventative strategies seems to be indicated by the significant number of black children entering care on a voluntary basis, the evidence appears to suggest a lack of access to and use of these services. The opposite appears to be the case in terms of access to compulsory care. For children who have one black parent and one white there is little disagreement about their over-representation. For children whose parents are both black the national studies appear to be in disagreement with the local studies, which do show over-representation. There is also some evidence that out of all black children, those of Asian origin may be under-represented.

In terms of the characteristics of black children who come into care, all the studies show that the majority of black children in care or admitted to care were under the age of five. Furthermore, there is little evidence of significant numbers of black teenagers entering care. Barn's is the only study that explores gender differences, noting that black girls were more likely than white girls to be admitted into care. In terms of family circumstances Barn provides the greatest amount of detail, noting the dominance of female lone parent households with a significant number of women in white collar and skilled manual occupations.

All the work that examines legal status note black children's entry into care through the voluntary route (Section 2 of the 1980 Children Act), and this was significantly so in comparison to white children. However, Barn suggests that within a short period of being in care black children were likely to experience a change in legal status which would see them move from their voluntary status to compulsory status: in effect becoming more like their white counterparts.

The studies also show that although there is evidence of the continued presence of black children in residential establishments, it is clear that family placement is becoming the dominant form of care for black children, as it appears to be for most children. It is this move of black children from residential care in the 1970s (where black children were found to be 'languishing' with other 'special needs' or 'hard to place' children) to family placement that has been the other major research area. This work is increasingly considering the outcomes of these placements, not just where the child is placed.

The research reviewed, however, shows variability in outcome measure, amongst a range of other inconsistencies. This makes it a particularly arduous task to draw any conclusions from these studies regarding outcome, or to attach too much weight to them. However there is some suggestion that black children placed with black families will share similar (or better) outcomes to white children placed with white families. Furthermore, black children appear to benefit from the 'protective' factor of continued contact with their birth families (something that virtually all the studies agree upon), and black foster and adoptive parents may be particularly able in managing this. However children with one black and one white parent appear to be particularly at risk of unsuccessful outcomes, and are less likely to have the protection of continued contact with the birth family.

Black elders

The 1991 Census suggests that the number of black people of pensionable age is just over 164,000. This is a rise of 168 per cent on the 1981 figure of just 61,000. The studies reviewed here, though small scale and local, demonstrate that this group of black people have considerable health and social care needs. While the evidence on intensity is sketchy, it is clear that in the inability to perform some basic tasks affects a comparatively younger group of black older people than white older people.

The evidence also demonstrates that black older people are likely to have lower levels of income than white older people. Black older people are also more likely to live in poorer housing and lack basic amenities. Indeed Owen in his analysis of the 1991 Census notes that the fact that 'more than half of all households headed by persons from each of the three black ethnic groups do not possess a car compared to a third of white headed households': this strongly indicates that black households have much lower income levels than white households. Further their receipt of pensions is low since they fall short on all the criteria which generally lead to better pensions: type of occupation; stability of employment; and final salary. For the majority, therefore, income in older age is made up significantly by means-tested benefits.

Though the proportion of 'pensioner only' households is low amongst black older people, the family and household structure of black older people is not homogenous. The evidence suggests that while pensioner only or lone pensioner households are rare in Bangladeshi communities, these are closer to white levels for the black Caribbean communities. However a higher proportion of black older people do live in multi-generational households. Nevertheless studies suggest that this does not mean that they have no need for care and that their needs are being met by the extended family and network. Studies show that in some of these multi-generational families other family members are unwilling to care for their elders, while in others they are severely restricted in the care that they can provide because of lack of resources, lack of services or sometimes the inappropriateness of services. Many studies therefore suggest that often in terms of black elders provision is about containment rather than care.

Common to all of the studies and research reviewed here is the low level of knowledge about services and under-use by black older people. Issues relating to accessibility, appropriateness and communication have been identified as the main barriers to use of services.

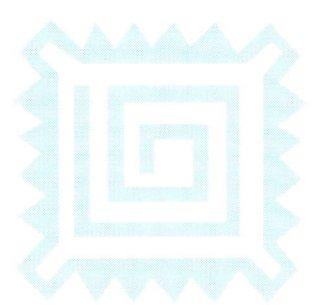

Mental health

Western definitions of mental health (well-being and illness) are at the heart of the debate to explain the differing experiences between black and white people of mental health services. If the western diagnosis of mental illness is accepted, then over-representation of black people in the 'harder end' of mental health services is explained by higher rates of psychosis (in particular schizophrenia). If, however, the application of western diagnosis to black communities is doubted and rejected then other factors - most importantly racism - explain this situation. Importantly racism does not only explain mis-diagnosis but highlights the presence of black people in the most controlling regimes, at the same time as their absence from more supportive services such as counselling.

Whether or not black people are in the mental health system as a result of greater likelihood of illness or because of discrimination, it is clear that they are certainly over-represented in the 'harder end': compulsorily detained under a legal order. This is particularly so for those of Afro-Caribbean origin. The evidence varies as to whether this is only so for first generation (migrant) Afro-Caribbeans or second generation (British born) Afro-Caribbeans. Also there is some variance in terms of age and gender. However over-representation of Afro-Caribbeans is almost universally accepted. The evidence for

Asians is contradictory, with some studies suggesting similar patterns
to white people, while others demonstrate over-representation for
Indians or Pakistanis or young Asian men. However, studies that have
examined this age group have shown Asians are less likely to be diagnosed as schizophrenic then their Afro-Caribbean counterparts.

This over-representation in compulsory detention appears to also
mean that black people are over-represented in the most controlling
regimes: secure units. Importantly, however, there are no national
figures available to challenge or confirm the local studies.
Interestingly, evidence from Cope (1989) suggests that those of Afro-
Caribbean origin in secure units are more likely to have been charged
with less serious offences than their white counterparts. Furthermore,
they are less likely to be described as aggressive than their white
counterparts in secure units.

All black people appear to have some difficulty in accessing
counselling, including psychotherapy. This is probably due to a combination of factors: they are sent into that part of the system which is
more likely to use physical treatment; the counselling service is either
inadequate or inappropriate to their needs; or they are unaware of
the availability of these services. However when these services are
available and appropriate there is evidence of use and a feeling
amongst black people that they are benefiting.

Disability

In reviewing the evidence of incidence and prevalence of social care
needs of black disabled people, it is important to note that these
studies demonstrate that there remains the unresolved issue of how
to define disability: whether to use a medical model or one that draws
attention to how society disables. Having acknowledged this difficulty,
the research studies reviewed here suggest that there are few instances
where the prevalence of disability (or long term limiting illness) is
lower in black communities than the white population when taking
age into account. The national evidence for higher rates is unclear.
However smaller scale or local studies do suggest higher rates
(particularly for older people), but this may vary in terms of the
constituent parts of black communities.

Those studies that identify higher rates of disability in black
communities suggest that this is true of both physical and sensory
disabilities as well as learning disabilities. Often pathological explanations have been forwarded to explain some of these higher rates.
However, while some research has suggested that congenital rubella
syndrome and first cousin marriages may be in part the cause, there
is evidence to show that it is unlikely to fully explain the higher levels

of disability amongst black people. Socio-economic factors and issues relating to access to and delivery of services are more likely to impact: factors such as money, housing, education. All these factors also appear to play a part in understanding disability levels in the white community.

While the exact rate of disability in black communities as well as the causes remain open to debate, there is sufficient evidence to demonstrate the existence of disability amongst black communities and that these disabilities are accompanied with social care needs. The studies reviewed further show that access to and knowledge of services is low amongst both black disabled people and their carers.

Some studies also suggest that the experience of disability is different for black disabled people than their white counterparts. Black disabled people have to contend with discrimination and disadvantages associated with their disability and as a result of racism. However, care must be taken with viewing black disabled people's lives in terms of competing or cumulative oppressions. The reality is more likely to be different situations bringing different oppressions to prominence, as well as highlighting the importance of past experiences of individuals. The concept of multiple oppression appears to be more appropriate than concepts of 'double' or 'triple' jeopardy'.

Carers

The small number of studies on informal care within black communities show that the mainstay of this care are predominantly women. Furthermore, that caring is not a new phenomenon, with many of these women having been principle carers for some years. Also that the needs of black carers are numerous, ranging from education on health, diet and care, to support with caring. Importantly, just as is the case for some white carers, carers in black communities appear to be unsupported and isolated. This is often exacerbated by communication difficulties and the lack of sensitive and appropriate services. Service provision continues to remain ethnocentric, geared to meeting the needs of the white majority. Further, there is evidence to show that black carers are often more severely affected by the problems of poverty and bad housing.

Studies also explode the myth of 'black people looking after their own'. It appears that the higher proportion of multi-generational households in black communities is taken as evidence of an existence of caring relationships. Additionally, there is evidence that the extended network of family support is not readily achievable in Britain because of migration patterns which have tended to divide families. Finally, studies also suggest that simply living in a large family does not always mean that support is available and that the needs of those being cared for and those caring are adequately met.

Using the research evidence

Much of the research presented here raises issues of comparability within their own 'subject areas'. It is therefore potentially dangerous to attempt to draw out themes across all the subject areas. Nevertheless, it is worth highlighting some of these themes as they impact on how the research evidence may be used to bring about change both in the provision of social care, and in the lives of black service users.

Needs

The literature on identifying needs already highlights the importance of value judgements in this process (see the discussion in chapter 1 page 6). Attempting to identify the social and health care needs of black communities in England probably epitomises this point. A constant theme in this review - whether we consider the needs of black children and their families, or of black elders, or those who may have mental health problems - is that the values brought to considering the problems black communities face will impact on how their needs are defined as well as how to respond to them. It is unlikely that the differences in values in some instances will ever be resolved: for example those who explain higher compulsory detention of black people under the 1983 Mental Health Act as a product of higher rates of psychotic illness, and those who suggest that this is reflective of the operation of discriminatory practice in assessing black people's mental state. Nevertheless, it is important to recognise that all these positions do have a value base. Similarly, social care providers who have attempted to develop and provide appropriate services have also been shown to make value judgements as to what the needs are and how they should be met: decisions to set up interpreting and translation services or to treat all disabled people the same are some examples.

Doyal and Gough have criticised those involved in promoting the rights of people who have experienced discrimination for at times arguing that all needs are relative and suggesting that some needs may only be identifiable by those who have experienced that discrimination: see their discussion of Shah (1986) in Doyal and Gough, 1991:15. Their criticisms do highlight the imperative of ensuring that taking account of discrimination does not mean the creation of a situation where all actions are explained (and excused) because of the different values various people or groups may have. Nevertheless any examination of what is a good service (or a bad service) must explore the judgements social care providers have made in deciding whether a particular problem faced by black communities is a need, and that this is the way they intend to respond to it.

The evidence reviewed also suggests that those agencies who respond by saying 'we treat everyone the same' have either not considered the needs of black communities or have taken a decision to ignore them. Furthermore, the 1989 Children Act and the 1990 NHS and Community Care Act place a responsibility on social care providers to identify the needs of particular population groups and individuals in order to plan the delivery of services as well as to tailor services to particular individuals. Evidence from this review often draws on research completed before the implementation of either Act. However it does act as a signpost: agencies that do not make a specific effort to analyse the needs of black communities are not making any serious effort to respond to the needs of these communities.

Assessment

As the process of assessment becomes more formalised (both by developments in practice as well as through the requirements of the 1989 Children Act and the 1990 NHS and Community Care Act) its importance appears to have grown. However this review suggests that assessment has always been crucial in the interaction between black communities and social care providers. Assessment that has viewed some black families as dysfunctional, while other black families are viewed as insular and able to meet their own social care needs, appears to exacerbate the problems of black people rather than ameliorating them. We have the contrasting pictures of black elderly people not using home care and home help services, apparently because this care is being provided for them by their families; while very young black children are over-represented in care because of their family's inability to provide adequate care.

Once again the evidence is contentious, and it is likely that all we can safely conclude at present is that the assessment process (the information recorded and given to clients, how information is collected and the decisions that result) must be shown not to be making judgements based on stereotypical views of black family life. However if social care is to contribute to black people living full and active lives, assessment will have to do more: it will have to demonstrate how it is leading to black people being allocated appropriate services. Any inspection would then have to consider how well this has been achieved.

Information

The burst of data that has resulted from the inclusion of an ethnic group question in the 1991 Census is one aspect of another constant theme in this review: information. Lack of information has been seen as an explanation for both the failure to consider whether black communities have specific social care needs as well as the failure to provide appropriate services. Furthermore, some of the controversy that has surrounded research on black communities has been the result of questions with regard to the quality of information available: the 1981 Census for example. Importantly, our review shows that information has been and is a problem for black communities also. The failure to use some services is associated with a lack of information about their availability and how to access them. This may have led in some circumstances to black people only coming to the attention of social care agencies when the situation requires significant intervention (such as compulsory detention under the 1983 Mental Health Act), whereas earlier intervention might have prevented the situation deteriorating.

However, response to the information needs of social care agencies and black communities appears to be limited. The presentation of results from the 1991 Census often appears to be fuelled by the fact that the information is there, rather than as a result of a consideration of what this information can be used for. In similar fashion, translated material is made available with little consideration of the role of information in providing appropriate services and often excludes some black communities (particularly the Afro-Caribbean community). If better communication with black communities plays a part in providing better services, then social care agencies must exploit the information resources available to them with this in mind, and must also make information available with this intention.

Monitoring

As social care agencies begin to be increasingly required to provide a purposeful service, their ability to identify what the outcomes of their interventions are is drawing attention. This review has suggested that in many instances it is still not possible to achieve what is probably the first stage of this process: identifying who is getting which service. The non-availability of ethnicity based information for those people in secure units run by the Special Hospitals Authority, and the failure to implement the Department of Health draft circular on recording the ethnicity of children in 'the public care', are a couple of national examples of this problem. Although the national picture has been improved recently with the beginning of ethnic record keeping for all in-patients, we are still some way from being able to say who gets which service. At a local level a similar situation exists, with evidence that even for those departments that do have ethnic record keeping and monitoring systems, the system is likely to be little more than the ability to record ethnic origin in a computer field.

This review demonstrates that the debate about outcomes for black people who receive (or do not receive) services from social care agencies is only in its infancy. But its development is likely to be severely hindered without reference to ethnicity information. Various studies have detailed individual acts of racism and, by way of contrast, the provision of appropriate services. Nevertheless for there to be any exploration of whether these result from the actions of individual workers or the actions of organisations, there must be availability of ethnicity based information for all services.

Furthermore, without this information monitoring, review or inspections exercises will only be able comment on an individualised basis. The recent Ritchie (1994) report on the care and treatment of Christopher Clunis demonstrates this most starkly. This suggested that no examples of prejudice or discrimination were found (Ritchie et al, 1994:4), yet the detailed recording of Christopher's experience of hospitals, discharge from hospitals, medication, and community services, echoed the experiences of other black people (see Harris, 1994; Reed, 1994). But without some way of examining whether the experience of Clunis was an individual experience or part of a pattern the debate remains open, with doubts expressed about how effectively Ritchie's recommendations will ameliorate this situation for black people.

Similarly, without this information it will be impossible to comment on comparative performance. An essential element of the monitoring, review or inspection process is the ability to identify those care providers that are doing well and those that need to make improvements. Once again, without ethnicity based information this will not be possible.

Inspection
While much of the research evidence reviewed here shows areas of concern that could legitimately be deemed priorities for inspection by social care agencies or the Social Services Inspectorate, a more general question must be considered first: should there be specific inspections of services being delivered to black communities, or should these concerns be integrated into 'mainstream' inspections? If the research reviewed here is seen as evidence of the value of the two different approaches then the answer appears to be that both approaches are necessary. Setting aside the many caveats raised about the studies considered by this review, it is the case that the specific

inquiries into the services that black communities are receiving (or not receiving) appear to be particularly able in identifying how social care agencies are responding to the social care needs of black communities. In similar fashion, those (few) studies that place the black communities' experiences of a particular service in the context of a service as a whole are useful because they allow the experiences of various communities to be compared and contrasted.

In some senses the dichotomy is false, because many of the studies specifically looking at the experience of black communities do try and place their evidence in the context of the whole service. But this still suggests that in the focusing and targeting of inspection activity, both approaches are required. Some inspection activity will have to focus specifically on services to black communities, while others will have to assess services to black communities as part of a wider assessment. Both approaches will have to be conscious of some of the pitfalls: for example when focusing on services being delivered to black communities there is been a tendency in the studies to concentrate on areas with 'high' black populations to the exclusion of some areas where black communities are more isolated, and as a consequence may be more vulnerable in times of distress. In addition, regardless of the approach adopted it is clear from this review that it is no longer adequate for inspections to ignore the experience of black communities in either collecting data or their presentation.

To conclude, the themes that emerge from this review suggest that in considering focusing and targeting of inspection activity the attention has to be paid to how needs are identified, how assessment is carried out, what information is available to social care providers and black communities and, finally, whether and how services are monitored. In addition, for the foreseeable future, at times inspection will have to focus specifically on black communities, and on other occasions include these as part of wider investigations.

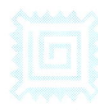

Bibliography

Social care bibliographies

Amin, K, Fernandes, M and Gordon, P (1988) **Racism and Discrimination in Britain: A Select Bibliography** 1984-87, Runnymede Trust.

Gordon, P and Klug, F (1984) **Racism and Discrimination in Britain: A Select Bibliography** 1970-83, Runnymede Trust.

Institute for Race Relations (1993) **Resource Directory on 'Race' and Racism in Social Work**, IRR.

Johnson, M R D (1985) **Race and Care An indexed bibliography of material on multi-cultural welfare services**, Centre for Research in Ethnic Relations.

Shaw, M (1988) **Family Placement for Children in Care: A guide to the literature, BAAF.**

Shaw, M (1994) **A Bibliography of Family Placement Literature**, BAAF.

Abrahams, C and Mungall, R (1992) **Runaways: Exploding the Myths**, National Children's Home.

Ahmad, B (1989) Child care and ethnic minorities, in Kahan, B **Child Care Research, Policy and Practice**, pp153-168, Open University.

Ahmad, W I U et al (1989) Health of British Asians: a research review, **Community Medicine**, 11, pp49-56.

Akinsola, H A A and Fryers, T (1986) A comparison of patterns of disability in severely mentally handicapped children of different ethnic origins, **Psychological Medicine**, Vol 16, pp127-133.

Almas, T (1992) After recruitment: putting the preparation and training of Asian carers on the agenda, **Adoption and Fostering** Volume 16, No 3, pp25 - 29.

Asian Disability Advisory Project Team (ADAPT) (1993) **Asian and Disabled: A study into the needs of Asian people with disabilities in the Bradford Area**, Barnardos Keighley Project and The Spastics Society.

Askham, J (1992) Health and social service provision: potential users amongst Black and minority ethnic elderly people, in Morton, J (1992) **Ageing Update: Conference Proceedings - Recent Research on Services for Black and Minority Ethnic Elderly People**, Institute of Gerontology, pp17 - 23.

Askham, J (1992) Health and social services provision: the service providers, in Morton, J (1992) **Ageing Update: Conference Proceedings - Recent Research on Services for Black and Minority Ethnic Elderly People**, Institute of Gerontology, pp9 -16.

Askham, J, Henshaw, L and Tarpey, M (1995) **Social and Health Authority Services for Elderly People from Black and Minority Ethnic communities**, HMSO.

Atkin, K and Rollings, J (1991) **Community Care in a Multi-racial Britain: A critical review of the literature**, HMSO, pp9 - 11.

Atkin, K et al (1989) **Asian Elders' Knowledge and Future Use of Community Social and Health Services**, University of Birmingham, Community Care Project, No22.

Badat, H and Whall-Roberts, D (1994) **Bridging the Gap**, RNID.

Bailey, J (1993) 1991 Census results - for local authority districts in Great Britain, **Population Trends** No 73, pp8 -17, HMSO/OPCS.

Balarajan, R and Botting, B (1989) Perinatal mortality in England and Wales: variations by mother's country of birth, **Health Trends**, Vol 21, pp79-84.

Balarajan, R, Yuen, P and Soni Raleigh, V (1989) Ethnic differences in general practice consultations, **British Medical Journal**, 299, 6705, pp958-960.

Balarajan, R and Bulusu, L (1990) Mortality among immigrants in England and Wales, 1979-83, in Britton, M (ed) (1990), **Mortality and Geography: A Review in the Mid-1980s, England and Wales**, pp103-121, HMSO.

Banks, N (1992) Techniques for direct identity work with black children, **Adoption and Fostering**, Vol 16, No 3, pp19- 24.

Barker, J (1984) **Black and Asian People in Britain**, Age Concern.

Barn, R (1990) Black children in local authority care: admission patterns, **New Community**, Vol 16, No 2, pp229-246.

Barn, R (1993) **Black Children in the Public Care System**, Batsford.

Batta, I, McCullogh, J and Smith, N (1975) A study of juvenile delinquency among Asians and half-Asians, **British Journal of Criminology**, Vol 15 no 1, pp32-42.

Batta, I and Mawby R (1981) Children in local authority care: a monitoring of racial differences, in Bradford, **Policy and Politics**, Vol 9, No 2, pp137-149.

Baxter, C (1989) **Cancer Support and Ethnic Minority and Migrant Work Communities**, Cancerlink.

Baxter, C, Poonia, K and Ward, L (1990) **Double Discrimination**, Kings Fund Centre/CRE.

Baylies, C, Law, I and Mercer, G (1993) **The Nature of Care in a Multi-racial Community: Summary report of an investigation of the support for Black and ethnic minority persons after discharge from psychiatric hospitals in Bradford and Leeds**, University of Leeds.

Bebbington, A and Miles, J (1990) The supply of foster families for children in care, **British Journal of Social Work**, Vol. 20, pp283-307.

Bebbington, A, and Miles, J (1989) The background of children who enter local authority care, **British Journal of Social Work** Vol. 19, pp349 -368.

Begum, N (1995) Care management and assessment from an anti-racist perspective, **Social Care Research Findings**, no 65, Joseph Rowntree Foundation.

Begum, N (1994) Mirror, mirror on the wall, in Begum, N, Hill, M and Stevens, A **Reflections: The View of Black Disabled People on Their Lives and Community Care**, CCETSW.

Begum, N (1992) **Something To Be Proud Of: The lives of Asian disabled people and carers in Waltham Forest**, Race Relations Unit and Disability Unit, London Borough of Waltham Forest.

Begum, N, Hill, M and Stevens, A (1994) **Reflections: The View of Black Disabled People on Their Lives and Community Care**, CCETSW.

Beliappa, J (1991) **Illness or Distress? Alternative Models of Mental Health**, Confederation of Indian Organisations.

Berridge, D and Cleaver, H (1987) **Foster Home Breakdown**, Basil Blackwell.

Berry, S, Lee, M and Griffiths, S (1981) **Report and Survey of West Indian Pensioners in Nottingham**, Nottingham Social Services Department.

Bhalla, A and Blakemore, K (1981) **The Elderly of the Minority Ethnic Groups**, All Faiths for One Race.

Bhat, A, Carr-Hill, R and Ohri, S (1988) **Britains Black Population - A New Perspective**, Radical Statistics Race Group.

Bhopal, R S and Donaldson, L J (1988) Health education for ethnic minorities - current provision and future direction, **Health Education Journal**, 47, 4, pp137-40.

Bhrolchain, M (1990) The ethnicity question for the 1991 Census, **Ethnic and Racial Studies**, Vol. 13, No 4, October.

Biehal, N, Clayden, J, Stein, M and Wade, J (1995) Black young people: experiences and identities, in Biehal, N, Clayden, J, Stein, M and Wade, J **Moving On - Young People and Leaving Care Schemes**, pp117 - 129, HMSO.

Biehal, N, Clayden, J, Stein, M and Wade, J (1995) **Moving On - Young People and Leaving Care Schemes**, HMSO.

Blakemore, K (1983) Ageing in the inner city: a comparison of old blacks and old whites, in Jerrome, D (ed) **Ageing in Modern Society**, Croom Helm.

Blakemore, K (1982) Health and illness among the elderly of minority ethnic groups living in Birmingham: some new findings, **Health Trends**, Vol 14, August, pp69-72.

Blakemore, K (1989) Does age matter? The case of old age in minority ethnic groups, in Bytheway, B et al (eds) **Becoming and Being Old: Sociological Approaches to Later Life**, Sage.

Blakemore, K and Boneham, M (1994) **Age, Race and Ethnicity: A Comparative Approach**, Open University Press.

Bolton, P (1984) Management of compulsory admitted patients to a high security unit, **International Journal of Social Psychiatry**, Vol 30, pp77-84.

Boneham, M A (1989) Ageing and ethnicity in Britain: the case of elderly Sikh women in a Midlands town, **New Community**, pp447-459.

Bourne, J (1981) Cheerleaders and ombudsmen: a sociology of race relations in Britain, **Race and Class**, 21, pp331-352.

Bowl, R and Barnes, M (1990) Race, racism and mental health social work: implications for local authority policy and training, **Research, Policy and Planning**, Vol 18, No 2, pp12 - 18.

Bowling, B (Sept 1990) **Elderly People from Ethnic Minorities: A Report on Four Projects**, Age Concern Institute of Gerontology, Kings College London.

Bowling, B (1992) Helping the community to care: four innovatory projects, in Morton, J (1992) **Ageing Update: Conference Proceedings - Recent**

Research on Services for Black and Minority Ethnic Elderly People, Institute of Gerontology, pp5-8.

British Association of Social Workers (BASW) Special Interest Group on Services for People with a Mental Handicap (1987), **Newsletter**, No 7, January.

Brown, C (1984) **Black and White Britain: The Third PSI Survey**, Gower.

Brozovic, M, Davies, S, and Henthorn, J (1989) Haematological and clinical aspects of sickle cell disease in Britain, in Cruickshank, J and Beevers, D, pp103-113.

Bulsara, S (1988) Services for all, **Carelink**, 6, 6.

Butt, J, Gorbach, P and Ahmad, B (1991) **Equally Fair? A report on social services departments' development, implementation and monitoring of services for the black and minority ethnic community**, NISW. (Re-printed by HMSO in 1994)

Butt, J (1994) **Same Service or Equal Services? The second report on social services departments' development, implementation and monitoring of services for the black and minority ethnic community**, HMSO.

Butt, J (1994b) Exploring and using the black resource in research, **Research, Policy and Planning**, Vol 12 no 2, pp9-12.

Butt, J (1996) Race equality: understanding recent evidence of child abuse and neglect in black families, in **Community Care Research Matters**, April-October 1996, pp50-52.

Cameron, E et al (1988) **Black Old Women, Disability and Health Carers**, Health Services Research Centre, University of Birmingham.

Carby, H (1982) White woman listen! Black feminism and the boundaries of sisterhood, Hall, S(Ed) in **The Empire Strikes Back**, Hutchinson.

Carrington, L (1995) The cost of caring, **Community Care**, 9-15 March.

Chakrabarti, M and Cadman, M (1994) **Survey of Needs of Minority Ethnic Elders and Carers for Social Work Support in Tayside**, Department of Social Work, University of Strathclyde.

Charles, M, Rashid, S and Thoburn, J Thoburn, (1992) The placement of black children with permanent new families, **Adoption and Fostering** Vol. 16, No 3, pp13 - 19.

Charlton, J, Wallace, M and White, I (1994) Long term illness: results from the 1991 census, **Population Trends**, No 75, Spring, pp19 - 25.

Cheetham, J (1981) Positive discrimination in social work, **New Community**, Vol 5, Part 1, p28.

Chiu, S (1989) Chinese elderly people: no longer a treasure at home, **Social Work Today**, Vol 2, No 48, pp15-17.

Clarke, P et al (1993) **Improving Mental Health Practice**, Northern Curriculum Development Project, CCETSW.

Cochrane, R (1977) Mental illness in immigrants to England and Wales: an analysis of mental hospital admissions, 1971, **Social Psychiatry**, Vol 12.

Cocking, I and Athwal, S (1990) A special case for treatment, **Social Work Today**, Vol 21, No. 2, pp12-13.

Cohen, R et al (1992) **Hardship Britain: Being Poor in the 1990s**, CPAG.

Cole, J (1990) **The Needs of Elderly Black People, Carers and Black People with Disabilities**, Lewisham Social Services, London Borough of Lewisham.

Commission for Racial Equality (1984a) **Race and Council Housing in Hackney: Report of a Formal Investigation**, CRE.

Commission for Racial Equality (1984b) **Race and Housing in Liverpool: A Research Report**, CRE.

Commission for Racial Equality (1989) **Racial Discrimination in Liverpool City Council: Report of a Formal Investigation into the Housing Department**, CRE.

Confederation of Indian Organisations (1986) **Double Bind: To Be Disabled and Asian**, CIO.

Confederation of Indian Organisations (1987) **Asians and Disabilities**, CIO.

Coombes, M, Raybould, S, Wong, C and Openshaw, S (1995) Part 1. Towards an index of deprivation: a review of alternative approaches, in **1991 Deprivation Index: A Review of Approaches and a Matrix of Results**, HMSO.

Cope, R (1989) The compulsory detention of Afro-Caribbeans under the Mental Health Act, **New Community**, Vol. 15, No.3, pp343 - 356.

Cope, R and Ndegwa, D (1990) Ethnic differences in admissions to a regional secure unit, **Journal of Forensic Psychiatry**.

Cross, M (1991) Editorial, **New Community** Vol 17, No 3, pp307-311.

Curtis, S (1989) **Juvenile Offending - Prevention Through Intermediate Treatment**, Batsford.

De'Ath, E (1989) Families and children, in Kahan, B (ed) **Child Care Research, Policy and Practice**, Open University, pp30-54.

Department of Environment (1979) **English Housing Condition Survey 1976: Part 2 Report of the Social Survey**, Housing Survey Report, No 11, DOE.

Department of Environment (1991) **English Housing Condition Survey**, DOE.

Department of Health (1992) **Patterns and Outcomes in Child Placement: Messages from Current Research and Their Implications**, HMSO.

Derby Commission for Racial Equality (nd) **Ethnic Elderly of Derby**, Derby CRE, Derbyshire Social Services and Derbyshire College of Higher Education.

Divine, D (ed) (1991) **One Small Step Towards Racial Justice**, CCETSW.

Donaldson, L (1986) Health and social status of elderly Asians: a community survey, **British Medical Journal**, 293, 25 October.

Donaldson, L J and Odell, A (1984) **Aspects of the Health and Social Services Needs of Elderly Asians in Leicester: A Community Survey**, University of Leicester.

Donovan, J (1984) Ethnicity and race: a research review, **Social Science and Medicine**, 19, 7.

Doyal, L and Gough, I (1991) **The Theory of Human Need**, Macmillan.

Driedger, L and Chappell, N L (1987) **Ageing and Ethnicity: Towards an Interface**, Butterworths.

Ebrahim, S et al (1991) Prevalence and severity of morbidity among Asian elders: a controlled comparison, **Family Practice**, 8, pp57-62.

Eribo, L (1991) **The Support You Need: Information for Carers of Afro-Caribbean Elderly People**, Kings Fund Centre.

Evandrou, M (1994) Review of recent studies, **Journal of Social Policy**, Vol 23, No 4, pp599-601.

Evers, H, Badger, F, Cameron, E and Atkin, K (1988) **Community Care Project Working Papers**, Department of Social Medicine, University of Birmingham.

Farrah, M (1986) **Black Elders in Leicester: An action research report on the needs of black elderly people of African descent from the Caribbean**, Leicester Social Services Department.

Fenton, S (1986) **Race, Health and Welfare: Afro-Caribbean and South Asian People in Central Bristol: Health and Social Services**, Department of Sociology, University of Bristol (unpublished report).

Fenton, S (1987) **Ageing Minorities: Black People As They Grow Old in Britain**, Commission for Racial Equality.

Fenton, S and Sadiq, A (1990) **South Asian Women in UK and Depression** - Paper presented at the conference British Sociological Association (Medical Sociology subgroup), Edinburgh.

Finkelhor, D and Barron, L (1986) High risk children, in Finkelhor, D **A Sourcebook on Child Sexual Abuse**, SAGE.

First Key Leaving Care Advisory Service (1987) **A Study of Black Young People Leaving Care**, First Key, .

Flett, H, Henderson J, and Brown, B (1979) The practice of racial dispersal in Birmingham, 1969-1975, **Journal of Social Policy**, No 8, pp289-309.

Foren, R and Batta, I (1970) 'Colour' as a variable in the use made of a local authority child care department, **Social Work**, Vol 27 No 3, pp10-15.

Forrest, R and Gordon, D (1993) **People and Places: A 1991 Census Atlas of England**, SAUS.

Francis, E (1991) Mental health, antiracism and social work training, in Divine, D (ed) **One Small Step Towards Racial Justice**, CCETSW.

Francis, J (1993) Pressure group, **Community Care**, 18 March.

Fratter, J, Rowe, J, Sapford, D and Thoburn J (1991) **Permanent Family Placement - A Decade of Experience**, British Agencies for Adoption and Fostering.

Gambe, D et al (1992) **Improving Practice with Children and Families: A Training Manual**, Northern Curriculum Development Project, CCETSW.

Garbarino, J and Kostelny, K (1992) Child maltreatment as a community problem, **Child Abuse and Neglect**, Vol 16, pp455-464.

Gardner, R (1989) Consumer views, in Kahan, B (ed) **Child Care Research, Policy and Practice**, Open University, pp214-230.

Gardner, R (1992) Developing family support in local authority, in Gibbons, J (ed) **The Children Act 1989 and Family Support**, HMSO.

Gelfand, D E and Kutzik, A J (1979) **Ethnicity and Ageing: Theory, Research and Policy**, Springer.

Ghate, D and Spencer, L (1995) **The Prevalence of Child Sex Abuse in Britain**, HMSO.

Gibbons, J (ed) (1992) **The Children Act 1989 and Family Support: Principles into Practice**, HMSO.

Gibbons, J, Conroy, S and Bell, C (1995) **Operating the Child Protection System**, HMSO.

Gill, O and Jackson, B (1983) **Adoption and Race: Black, Asian and Mixed Race Children in White Families**, Batsford in association with BAAF.

GLAD (1987) **Disability and Ethnic Minority Communities: A Study in Three London Boroughs**, Greater London Association for Disabled People.

Glendenning, F and Pearson, M (1988) **The Black and Ethnic Minority Elders in Britain: Health Needs and Access to Services**, Health Education Authority and Centre for Social Gerontology, University of Keele.

Gorbach, P (1989) **Clarifying the Framework**, Research Unit, National Institute for Social Work (unpublished report).

Green, H (1988) **Informal Carers**, HMSO.

Grimley, M and Bhat, A (1989) Mental health, in Bhat, A, Carr-Hill, R and Ohri, S (eds) **Britain's Black Population**, Gower.

Grow, J L and Shapiro, D (1975) **Black Children White Parents: A Study of Transracial Adoption**, Research Centre, Child Welfare League of America Inc.

Gunaratnum, Y (1990) Asian carers, **Carelink**, Vol 11, No 6.

Harris, V (1994) **Review of the Report of the Inquiry into the Care and Treatment of Christopher Clunis - A Black Perspective**, Race Equality Unit, NISW, Critical Paper Series 1.

Haskey, J (1991) Estimated numbers and demographic characteristics of one parent families in Great Britain, **Population Trends** No 65, pp35 - 47.

Health Education Authority (1994) **Health and Lifestyles: Black and Minority Ethnic Groups in England**, Health Education Authority.

Heath, S and Dale, A (1994) The ethnic dimension, **Population Trends** No 77, pp5-13.

Hill, D and Penso, D (1995) **Opening Doors: Improving Access to Hospice and Specialist Palliative Care Services by Members of the Black and Ethnic Minority Communities**, National Council for Hospice and Specialist Palliative Care Services.

Hitch, P (1981) Immigration and mental health: local research and social explanations, **New Community**, Vol 9.

Hitch, P J and Clegg, P (1980) Modes of referral of overseas immigrant and native-born first admissions to psychiatric hospital, **Society, Science and Medicine**, Vol 14a, pp369-374.

Holzberg, G (1982) Ethnicity and ageing: anthropological perspectives on more than just the minority elderly, **Gerontologist**, Vol 22, No 3, pp249-257.

Home Office (1991) **Working Together Under the Children Act: A guide to arrangements for inter-agency co-operation for the protection of children from abuse**, HMSO.

Hunt, A (1978) **The Elderly at Home**, HMSO.

Husband, C (1991) 'Race', conflictual politics, and anti-racist social work: lessons from the past for action in the 90s, in Patel, N (ed) **Setting the Context for Change**, CCETSW.

Ineichen, B (1990) The mental health of Asians in Britain, **British Medical Journal**, Vol 300, pp1669-1670.

Ineichen, B (1989) Afro-Caribbeans and the incidence of schizophrenia: a review, **New Community**, Vol 15, No 3, pp335 - 341.

Jadeja, S and Singh, J (1993) Life in a cold climate, **Community Care**, 22 April.

Jones, A (1992) **Saying It Like It Is - Report of the Black and In Care Group**, Pankhurst Press.

Jones, A and Butt, J (1995) **Taking the Initiative**, NSPCC.

Jones, T (1993) **Britain's Ethnic Minorities**, Policy Studies Institute.

Joseph, G and Lewis, J (1981) **Common Differences**, South End Press.

Jowell, T et al (February 1990) **Action Project into the Needs of Carers in Black and Minority Ethnic Communities in Birmingham**, CCSAP/Kings Fund Centre.

Knapp, M, Baines, B and Fenyo, A (1988) Consistencies and inconsistencies in child care placements, **British Journal of Social Work**, Vol 18, pp107-130.

Knowles, C (1991) Afro-Caribbeans and schizophrenia: how does psychiatry deal with issues of race, culture and ethnicity? **Journal of Social Policy**, Vol 20, No 2, pp173-90.

Lalljie, R (1983) **Black Elders: A Discussion Paper**, Research Section, Social Services Department, Nottinghamshire County Council.

Lawrence, E (1982) In the abundance of water the fool is thirsty: sociology and black pathology, in Hall, S (ed) **The Empire Strikes Back**, Hutchinson.

Layzell, S and Lamb, B (1994) **Disabled in Britain: A World Apart**, Scope.

Lee, M (1987) **Sample Study of Black Families with a Mentally Handicapped Member**, Research Unit, Social Services Department, Nottinghamshire County Council.

Levin, E, Moriarty, J and Gorbach, P (1994) **Better for the Break**, HMSO.

Lewando-Hundt, G and Grant, L (1987) Studies of Black elders - an exercise in window dressing or the groundwork for widening provision, Coventry Survey, **Social Services Research**, Nos 5 and 6.

Littlewood R, K and Lipsedge M (1982) **Aliens and Alienists**, Penguin.

London Borough of Camden, **The Needs of Women Carers Whose First Language is not English**, Women's Unit, London Borough of Camden (Committee Report).

London Borough of Hackney (1985), **Child Care Policy - Ethnic Composition of Children in Care**, Social Services Race Relations Sub Committee, London Borough of Hackney (Committee Report).

London Borough of Lambeth (1981) **Black Children in Care: Report by the Director of Social Services**, London Borough of Lambeth.

Mama, A (1990) **The Hidden Struggle: Statutory and Voluntary Sector Responses to Violence Against Black Women in the Home**, Runnymede Trust.

Martin, J et al (1988) **OPCS Survey of Disability in Great Britain: The Prevalence of Disability Among Adults**, HMSO.

McAdam, L (1987) Racial analysis of children in care, **Social Services Research**, Vol 14, No 4, pp29-34 .

McAvoy, B R and Donaldson, L J (eds) (1990) **Health Care for Asians**, Oxford University Press.

McCalman, J A (1990) **The Forgotten People: Carers in Three Minority Ethnic Communities in Southwark**, Kings Fund Carers Unit.

McCormick, A, Rosenbaum, M and Fleming, D (1990) Socio-economic characteristics of people who consult their general practitioner, **Population Trends,** No 59, Spring.

McDonald, P (1991) Double discrimination must be faced now, **Disability Now**, March, 8.

McGovern, D and Cope, R (1987) The compulsory detention of males of different ethnic groups with special reference to offender patients, **British Journal of Psychiatry**, No 149, pp265-273.

McKillip, J (1987) **Need Analysis - Tools for the Human Services and Education**, Sage.

Mercer, K (1986) Racism and transcultural psychiatry, in Miller, P and Rose, N (eds) **The Power of Psychiatry**, Blackwell.

Miller, E et al (1987) Congenital rubella in babies of South Asian women in England and Wales: an excess and its causes, **British Medical Journal**, Vol 294, 21 March, pp737-739.

Moledina, S (1988) **Great Expectations: A Review of Services for Asian Elders in Brent**, Age Concern Brent.

Morris, J (1995) **Gone Missing: A research policy review of disabled children living away from their families**, Who Cares Trust.

NACRO (1991) **Race and Criminal Justice**, in NACRO Briefing Paper No 77, NACRO.

Neill, J and Williams, J (1992) **Leaving Hospital: Elderly People and Their Discharge to Community Care**, HMSO.

Norman, A (1985) **Triple Jeopardy: Growing Old in a Second Homeland**, Policy Studies in Ageing No 3, Centre for Policy on Ageing.

Nottinghamshire County Council (nd), **Annual Statistical Report 1990/91 - Children in Care**, Social Services Department, Nottinghamshire County Council.

Oliver, M (1992) Changing the social relations of research production, **Disability, Handicap and Society**, Vol 7 No 2 pp101-114.

OPCS (1992) **The Labour Force Survey 1990 and 1991**, HMSO

OPCS (1994) **Census Monitor**, OPCS.

OPCS (1988) **Social Trends 18**, HMSO.

Owen, C (1993) Using the labour force survey to etimate Britain's ethnic minority population, **Population Trends** No 72, pp18-23.

Owen, D (1992) **Ethnic Minorities in Great Britain: Settlement Patterns**, 1991 Census Statistical Paper No1, University of Warwick.

Owen, D (February 1993a) **Ethnic Minorities in Great Britain: Age and Gender Structure**, 1991 Census Statistical Paper No 2, University of Warwick.

Owen, D (March 1993b) **Ethnic Minorities in Great Britain: Economic Characteristics**, 1991 Census Statistical Paper No 3, University of Warwick.

Owen, D (April 1993c) **Ethnic Minorities in Great Britain: Housing and Family Characteristics**, 1991 Census Statistical Paper No 4, University of Warwick.

Owen, D (December 1993d) **Country of Birth: Settlement Patterns**, 1991 Census Statistical Paper No 5, University of Warwick.

Owen, D (February 1994a) **Black People in Great Britain: Social and Economic Circumstances**, 1991 Census Statistical Paper No 6, University of Warwick.

Owen, D (November 1994b) **South Asian People in Great Britain: Social and Economic Circumstances**, 1991 Census Statistical Paper No 7, University of Warwick.

Owen, D (December 1994c) **Chinese People and 'Other' Ethnic Minorities in Great Britain: Social and Economic Circumstances**, 1991 Census Statistical Paper No 8, University of Warwick.

Owen, D (1994d) Spatial variations in ethnic minority group population in Great Britain, **Population Trends**, No 78, pp23-33.

Owen, D (February 1995) **Irish Born People in Great Britain: Settlement Patterns and Socio-economic Circumstances**, 1991 Census Statistical Paper No 9, University of Warwick.

Parker, G and Lawton, D (1994) **Different Types of Care, Different Types of Carer: Evidence from the General Household Survey**, HMSO.

Patel, G (1994) **The Porth Project: A study of homelessness and running away amongst young black people in Newport, Gwent**, The Children's Society.

Patel, N (1990) A **'Race' Against Time? Social Services Provision to Black elders**, Runnymede Trust.

Pearson, M (1990) Ethnic differences in infant health, **Archives of Disease in Childhood**.

Pearson, R M (1986) The politics of ethnic minority health studies, in Rathwell, T and Phillips, D (eds) **Health, Race and Ethnicity**, Croom Helm.

Pharoah, C (1992) Primary health care: how well are users served?, in Morton, J (1992) **Ageing Update: Conference Proceedings - Recent Research** on Services for Black and Minority Ethnic Elderly People, Institute of Gerontology, pp24 - 32.

Pharoah, C (1995) **Primary Health Care for Elderly People from Black and Minority Ethnic Communities**, HMSO.

Phillips, M and Butt, J (1996) Enquiries into allegations: a black perspective, in Platt, D and Shemmings, D (Eds) **Making Enquiries into Alleged Child Abuse and Neglect**, Pennant.

Poonia, K and Ward, L (1990) Fair share of the care, **Community Care**, 11 January.

Population Statistics Division (1986) Ethnic minority populations in Great Britain, **Population Trends**, No 46 pp18-21.

Prime, R (1987) **Developing Social Services for Black and Ethnic Minority Elders in London: Overview Report and Action Plan**, Social Services Inspectorate, Department of Health and Social Security.

RADAR (1984) **Disability and Minority Ethnic Groups: A Factsheet of Issues and Initiatives**, Royal Association for Disability and Rehabilitation.

Rao, P S S and Inbaraj, S G (1980) Inbreeding effects on foetal growth and development, **Journal of Medical Genetics**, Vol 17, pp27-31.

Rathwell, T and Phillips, D (1986) (eds) **Health, Race and Ethnicity**, Croom Helm.

Reed, J (1994) **Review of Health and Social Services for Mentally Disordered Offenders and Others Requiring Similar Services Vol.6 Race, Gender and Equal Opportunities**, HMSO.

Rhodes, P J (1992) **Racial matching in Fostering**: The Challenge to Social Work Practice, Avebury.

Rickford, F (1994) Burden of care, **Community Care**, 21-27 July.

Ritchie, J, Dick, D and Lingham, R (1994) **The Report of the Inquiry into the Care and Treatment of Christopher Clunis**, HMSO.

Roberts, J (1991) **Sickle Cell Anaemia: The Hidden Disability Within the Black Community**, unpublished.

Robinson, C and Stalker, K (1992) **New Directions: Suggestions for Interesting Service Development in Respite Care**, Kings Fund Centre.

Robson, B, Bradford, M and Tye, R (1995) Part 2 A Matrix of deprivation in English Authorities, 1991, in **1991 Deprivation Index: A Review of Approaches and a Matrix of Results**, HMSO.

Rogers, A and Faulkner, A (1987) **A Place of Safety: MIND's Research into Police Referrals into the Psychiatric Services**, MIND.

Rosenthal, M et al (1988) Congenital hypothyroidism: increased incidence in Asian families, **Archives of Disease in Childhood**, Vol 63, pp790-793.

Rowe, J and Lambert, L (1973) **Children Who Wait: A Study of Children Needing Substitute Families**, Association of British Adoption Agencies.

Rowe, J, Cain, H, Hundleby, M and Keane, A (1984) **Long Term Foster Care**, Batsford in association with BAAF.

Rowe, J, Hundleby, M and Garnett, L (1989) **Child Care Now: A Survey of Placement Patterns**, BAAF.

Roys, P (1988) Social services, in Bhat, A, Carr-Hill R and Ohri, S (Eds) **Britain's Black Population - A New Perspective**, Radical Statistics Race Group, pp208 - 232.

Russell, P (1989) Handicapped children, in Kahan, B (ed) **Child Care Research Policy and Practice**, Open University, pp169-184.

Rwegellera, G G C (1980) Differential use of psychiatric services by West Indians, West Africans and English in London, **British Journal of Psychiatry**, Vol 137, pp428-432.

Sashidharan, S, P (1988) Conference Report by Greenwich Afro-Caribbean Alliance, **Mental Health in the Community**, pp44- 49.

Secretaries of State (1989) **Caring for People - Community Care in the Next Decade and Beyond**, HMSO.

Shah, R (1986) **Attitudes, Stereotypes and Service Provision**, Manchester Council for Community Relations.

Shaw, C (1988) Components of growth in the ethnic minority population, **Population Trends**, No 52.

Sheppard, D (1995) **Learning the Lessons: Mental health inquiry reports published in England and Wales between 1969 - 1994 and their recommendations for improving practice**, The Zito Trust.

Sinclair, I, Parker, R, Leat, D and Williams, J (1990) **The Kaleidoscope of Care: A review of research on welfare provision for elderly people**, HMSO.

Smith, T (1992) Family centres, children in need and the Children Act 1989, in Gibbons, J (ed) **The Children Act 1989 and Family Support**, HMSO.

South Glamorgan County Council (1994) **County of South Glamorgan Social Care Plan 1994/5 - 1996/7 Part A**, SGCC.

South London Black Elderly Project (1995) **Findings from Three Years Work with African and Caribbean Elders in South London**, Wandsworth Black Elderly Project and Lambeth Black Elderly Luncheon Club.

Special Issue: Researching Disability (1992) **Disability, Handicap and Society**, Vol 7 Number 2.

Standing Conference of Ethnic Minority Senior Citizens (nd) **Making a Reality of Residential Care for Ethnic Minority Elders**, SCEMSC.

Stein, M, Rees, G and Frost, N (1994) **Running the Risk - Young People on the Streets of Britain Today**, The Children Society.

Stuart, O (1992) Race and disability: just a double oppression?, **Disability, Handicap and Society**, Vol 7 no 2, pp177-188.

Swarup, N (1992) **Equal Voice: Black Communities' Views on Housing, Health and Social Services**, Report No 22, Social Services Research and Information Unit.

Teague, A (1993) Ethnic group: first results from the 1991 Census, **Population Trends**, No 72, pp12-17.

Terry, P B et al (1985) Ethnic differences in congenital malformations, **Archives of Disease in Childhood**, Vol 60, pp866-868.

Timæus, I (1990) The fall in the number of children in care: a demographic analysis, 1979-1986, **Journal of Social Policy**, Vol 19, No 3, pp375-395.

Tirrito, T and Nathanson, I (1994) Ethnic differences in caregiving: adult daughters and elderly mothers, **AFFILIA: Journal of Women and Social Work**, Vol 19, No 1, Spring 1994.

Tizard, B and Phoenix, A (1989) Black identity and transracial adoption, **New Community**, Vol 15, No 3, pp427-437.

Townsend, P and Davidson, N, Whitehead, M and Black D (eds) (1988) **Inequalities in Health: The Black Report and the Health Divide**, Penguin.

Triseliotis, J (1989) Foster care outcomes: a review of key research findings, **Adoption and Fostering**, Vol 13, No 3, pp5-17.

Turnbull, A (1985) **Greenwich's Afro-Caribbean and South Asian Elderly People**, Planning and Research Section, London Borough of Greenwich.

Twigg, J (ed) (1992) **Carers: Research and Practice**, HMSO.

Ungerson, C (1990) **Gender and Caring**, Harvester Wheatsheaf.

Walby, C and Symons, B (1990) **Who Am I? Identity, Adoption and Human Fertilisation**, BAAF.

Walker, C (1987) How a survey led to providing more responsive help for Asian families, **Social Work Today**, Vol 19, No 7, pp12-13.

Walker, R and Ahmad, W I U (1994) Asian and black elders and community Care: A survey of care providers, **New Community**, Vol 20, No 4, pp636-646.

Wallace L (1991) **Black Carers - An Issues Paper**, Department of Social Studies, Selly Oak Colleges (unpublished).

Warburton, W R (July 1994) **Implementing Caring for People - Home and Away**, Department of Health.

Webb-Johnson, A (1991) **A Cry for Change - An Asian Perspective on Developing Quality Mental Health Care**, Confederation of Indian Organisations.

Whitehead, M (1987) **The Health Divides: Inequalities in Health in the 1980s, London**, London Education Authority.

Williams, J (1990) Elders from black and minority ethnic communities, in Sinclair, I et al (eds) **The Kaleidoscope of Care: A review of research on welfare provision for elderly people**, HMSO.

Wing, L (1969) Prevalence of different patterns of impairments in immigrants, in Wing, J K (ed) **Recent Research in Social Psychiatry**, MRC Social Psychiatry Unit, Institute of Psychiatry (unpublished report).

Wright, D (1992) Private fostering: public duty - private responsibility, **Adoption and Fostering**, Vol 16, No 3, pp30-34.

Appendix

1991 Census ethnic group full classification

Codes 0 to 6 are the pre-coded boxes in the question. Codes 7 to 34 were used for multi-ticking, and for 'writing in answers' given under 'Black Other' or 'Other ethnic group'

Code	Category
0	White
1	Black Caribbean
2	Black African
3	Indian
4	Pakistani
5	Bangladeshi
6	Chinese

Black Other: non-mixed origin

Code	Category
7	British
8	Caribbean Island, West Indies, or Guyana
9	North African, Arab, or Iranian
10	Other African countries
11	East African Asian or Indo-Caribbean
12	Indian sub-continent
13	Other Asian
14	Other answers

Black Other: mixed origin

Code	Category
15	Black/white
16	Asian/white
17	Other mixed

Other ethnic group: non-mixed origin

Code	Category
18	British - ethnic minority indicated

Code	Category
19	British - no ethnic minority indicated
20	Caribbean Island, West Indies, or Guyana
21	North African, Arab, or Iranian
22	Other African countries
23	East African Asian or Indo-Caribbean
24	Indian sub-continent
25	Other Asian
26	Irish
27	Greek (including Greek Cypriot)
28	Turkish (including Turkish Cypriot)
29	Other European
30	Other answers

Other ethnic group: mixed origin

Code	Category
31	Black/white
32	Asian/white
33	Mixed white
34	Other mixed

Ethnic group categories used for presenting results

The 35 codes above are grouped into 10 categories as follows:

White 0, 26-29, 33
Black Caribbean 1, 8, 20
Black African 2, 10, 22
Black other 7, 14, 15, 17
Indian 3
Pakistani 4
Bangladeshi 5

Chinese 6

Other groups
Asian 11-13, 23-25
Other 9, 16, 18, 19,
Non Asian 21, 30-32, 34

Notes

[1] The definition of this term as it relates to the Census is discussed on page 12. The ethnic group categories used to calculate these results are reproduced as an Appendix.

[2] As the estimates of the undercounting have appeared only recently, it is not always clear whether all the studies referred to here will have taken this into account.

[3] David Owen (1992) suggests that the 1991 Census did find one person from an ethnic minority community resident in the Scilly Isles.

[4] We must remain sceptical about the figures for 'Black-Other' for reasons detailed on page 18 of this chapter.

[5] Haskey (1991) presented a similar picture using the General Household Survey, pp38 and 39.

[6] Even though Charles et al (1992) are following up the work of Thoburn and Rowe (1988) and Fratter et al (1991), they add a new group of children that the previous studies did not consider.

[7] The Commission for Racial Equality has recently commissioned a study to explore this area.

[8] This question has been criticised, as have past attempts by OPCS to look at disability. In essence this question places the 'problem' at the door of those disabled rather than society, suggesting that it is the disabled person's fault that s(he) cannot, for example, use public transport rather than a failure on the part of public transport to meet her needs.

[9] In this context it is a phrase used by Karenga (1982, quoted by Divine, 1992) to explain the tension between seeing black people as passive victims or people who have managed to change and survive.

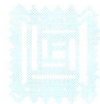

Index

Bold figures indicate a figure or table on that page

Camberwell, children with
  language impairment   91
Cameron, E.   104–5, 107–8
care, compulsory route   44–5;
  probability of entering **44**;
  voluntary route 44–**45**
care careers, black children
  and   39, 42–3
Caribbean   2, 12, 19; children in
  care system   41
Census (1981), black elderly
  populations and   68;
  information about black
  people   14, 124; numbers of
  Afro–Caribbeans in
  Britain   76, 116; Urban
  Priority Areas and   28 Census
  (1991)   3; age in ethnic
  minority groups   19–20; Black
  Caribbeans and Black
  Others   18; black people born
  in Britain   16; car ownership
  and black people   63, 118;
  ethnic group question   11, 13,
  15, 124; ethnic group
  classification   141; households
  with children under
  sixteen   33–4; housing and
  older black people   64;
  housing and tenure   24;
  limiting long term illness   56,
  85, 88, 90; low income levels
  for black people   63, 118;
  measure of 'family unit'   35;
  numbers of black elders   21,
  55, 118; overcrowding in
  households   25–6; people
  missing from   13; risk of
  deprivation and   27; single
  adult households   22, 59
Charles, M.   33, 48, 50–1
Charlton, J.   56, 88–90
children, mean number per
  family unit   **24**
Children Act (1980)   31, 46

Children Act (1989)   32, 35, 38,
  44, 123
children in care, age and gender
  of   42–3; ethnic origin of 31
  march (1990 and 1991)   **42**;
  family background   43–4; legal
  status of   44–5;
  outcomes   48–50; placement
  of   46–8
'Children entering care
  survey'   43
Children and Young Persons Act
  (1969)   31, 44
Chinese community, children in
  households   **24**;
  heterogeneous   15;
  households with
  pensioners   21, 56; limiting
  long term illness and   56, 89;
  pensioners   21–2, 55, 57;
  social services and older
  people   110
Cleaver, H.   48–9
Clunis, Christopher   80, 125
Cochrane, R.   75, 77
Cocking, I., Asian extended
  families   93, 107, 109, 111,
  114; Black carers   97–8, 105;
  sensory/learning disability   90
Cole, J.   110, 112–13
Commission for Racial Equality,
  discrimination and   26
Confederation of Indian
  Organisations (1986)   92–3, 96
congenital rubella, learning
  difficulties and   91–2, 120
containment, black elders
  and   53, 60–1, 70, 119
Coombes, M.   28, 116
Cope, R.   72, 74–8, 83, 120
counselling services, black people
  and   71, 81–2
Coventry, survey of black older
  people   64
Cross, M.   1, 81